By Christopher Dow

Fiction
Effigy
    Book I: Stroud
    Book II: Oakdale
The Books of Bob
    Devil of a Time
    Jumping Jehovah
The Clay Guthrie Mysteries
    The Dead Detective
    Landscape with Beast
    The Texas Troll Unlimited
Roadkill
The Werewolf and Tide, and other Compulsions

Nonfiction
Lord of the Loincloth (nonfiction novel)
Book of Curiosities: Adventures in the Paranormal
Occasional Pilgrimage: Essays on Film, Literature, and Other Matters
Living the Story: The Meandering, True, and Sometimes Strange
            Adventures of an Unknown Writer
    Vol.I: Growing Up Takes a Long Time
    Vol. II: Growing Old Takes Longer

Martial Arts
The Wellspring: An Inquiry into the Nature of Chi
Circling the Square: Observations on the Dynamics of Tai Chi Chuan
Elements of Power: Essays on the Art and Practice of Tai Chi Chuan
Alchemy of Breath: An Introduction to Chi Kung
Leaves on the Wind: A Survey of Martial Arts Literature (Vol. I-VI)

Poetry
City of Dreams
The Trip Out
Texas White Line Fever
Networks
A Dilapidation of Machinery
Puzzle Pieces: Selected Poems

Editor
The Abby Stone: The Poetry of Bartholo Dias
The Best of Phosphene
The Best of Dialog

LEAVES ON THE WIND

Volume IV

LEAVES ON THE WIND

A Survey of Martial Arts Literature

Volume IV

Overviews of the Internal Chinese Martial Arts
and books on
Xingyi/Yiquan, Bagua, Liuhebafa, Zimen Boxing,
Four-Section Boxing, Taiji Push Hands and Applications,
Wudang Weapons, and Narratives

CHRISTOPHER DOW

Phosphene Publishing Company
Temple, Texas

Leaves on the Wind: A Survey of Martial Arts Literature, Volume IV

© 2022 by Christopher Dow
ISBN: 978-1-7369307-8-6

Published by:
Phosphene Publishing Company
Temple, Texas, USA
phosphenepublishing.com

1.1

LEAVES ON THE WIND

volume IV

CONTENTS

Part III: Bagua

Part IV: Other Internal Styles

Part V: Push Hands & Applications

Part VI: Wudang Weapons

Part VII: Narratives

Appendix

PART I

Overviews of the
Internal Chinese Martial Arts

The Complete Works of Sun Lutang

by Sun Lutang
Translations by Paul Brennan
(*Brennan Translations*)

Throughout history, a fair number of people have created martial art styles. Many fewer have that martial art named for them rather than for characteristics of that art's method of movement. We are familiar with kung fu styles named for animals whose movements inspired these arts, such as Tiger, Praying Mantis, and Monkey. Some, like Aikido, which translates as "the Way of Combining Forces"[2], put together names that are amalgams of concepts. Other martial arts are named for people or families. Wing Chun, for example, is named for Yim Wing-chun, who learned the art from its founder, Abbess Ng Mui.[4] Sometimes names of martial art styles are created somewhat more poetically. Shotokan Karate was named for the dojo where its founder, Gichin Funakoshi, taught, and the dojo, in turn, was given that name as a combination of "Shoto," meaning waves of movement of pine needles blown by the wind (also Funakoshi's pen-name), and "kan," which meant "hall."[3]

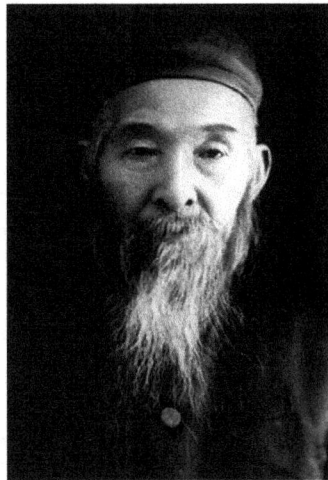

In a more straightforward sense, naming martial styles after their creators and their families seems to be a hallmark of Taiji. All five of the historically recognized Taiji styles are named for individuals or the families of their founders: Chen, Wu/Hao, Yang, Wu, and Sun. It is the founder of the latter who interests us here.

Sun Lutang, was born Sun Fuquan in Heibei, China in 1860. The name Lutang was given him by his Bagua teacher, Cheng Tinghua. Sun also learned Xingyi from Li Kuiyuan and Guo Yun-shen and already was an acknowledged high-level expert in both arts by the time he approached Taiji. It is interesting to note that the Taiji style he learned—Wu/Hao, which he picked up from Hao Wei-Chen—was, at the time and remains today, one of the lesser-practiced of Taiji's major styles. It wasn't long before Sun, whose abilities and understanding of the internal martial arts were profound, fused elements of Bagua, Xingyi, and Wu/Hao Taiji into his own—and perhaps the first—combined Taiji style: Sun Style.[1] Upon Sun Lutang's death, gatekeeping of the style was given to his second son, Sun Cunzhou, and his daughter, Sun Jianyun. Today, the International Sun Tai Chi Association is dedicated to preserving the knowledge of Sun Taiji as passed down through Sun Cunzhou's daughter, Sun Shurong. (See Volume VI of this series for a review of *Taiji Boxing* by Sun Jianyun.)

Sun Lutang wrote four books on specific internal martial arts, one book on basic internal martial arts philosophy and concepts, and four essays that cover additional general ground and that translator Paul Brennan has collected into a single volume. Apparently Sun also wrote a book on Bagua spear, though according to Brennan, it remains unpublished. The published works, in order of publication, are:

A Study of Xingyi Boxing (1915, trans. 2015, 140 pages)
A Study of Bagua Boxing (1917, trans. 2015, 69 pages)
A Study of Taiji Boxing (1921, trans. 2016, 88 pages)
Authentic Explanations of Martial Arts Concepts (1924, trans. 2013, 78 pages)
A Study of Bagua Sword (1927, trans. 2015, 46 pages)
Essays by Sun Lutang (trans. May 2015, 20 pages)
    "Discussing Distinctions Between the Internal & External Schools of Martial Arts" (1929)
    "Some Things I Have Been Told About Martial Arts" (1929)
    "My Opinions on the Origins of Chinese Martial Arts" (1930)
    "A Detailed Look at the Theories of Xingyi, Bagua, and Taiji" (1932)

I will review these books in a slightly different order. Please note that the number of pages refers not to the number in the original book but to the number in Brennan's translations when they are printed out.

A Study of Xingyi Boxing

A Study of Xingyi Boxing is Sun Lutang's first martial arts instruction manual, and it also is his longest. However, that length does not offer much in the way of historical or philosophical depth. Instead, the vast majority of the book is occupied by the form instruction section, which is highly detailed.

The book opens with prefaces by Zhao Heng and Ai Yukuan. Zhao's preface contains some amusing anecdotes regarding Bagua, but not much real substance. Ai's preface, on the other hand, does delve a bit deeper—though not too deeply—into the ideas that underlie all of the internal martial arts. He concludes that although Xingyi might be "called a 'boxing' art, it is actually a secret key for reenergizing one's life and a grand scheme for bringing longevity to the world. It is simultaneously martial and the Way."

Sun's own preface and a chapter called "General Comments" come next, and it is in these few pages that Sun opens to door to the Xingyi world. These pages contain a brief history of the art and its basic philosophy, but not much else. It does contain, though, this intriguing information:

> While once at Bai Xiyuan's home in Beijing, I got to see one of the Yue Fei manuals, not an original copy of course, but a handwritten copy made by someone in a later generation....I secretly made my own copy and then deeply studied it, going through it posture by posture until bit by bit I had built up the material to make this book.

Sun states that Yue Fei (1103-1142), a famous general and martial artist of the Song Dynasty, created Xingyi, though the historical record implies that the exact nature of Yue's martial style(s) is unknown. It is said that Yue studied at the Shaolin Monastery, and he is associated most closely with the creation of both Xingyi and Eagle Claw: the former for officers and the latter for enlisted men. The brief "General Comments" chapter also contains several important principles, such as emphasizing naturalness and the use of soft strength.

Sun is finished with all that by page eleven, and almost the entire remainder of the book is devoted to form instruction. If there was a paucity of information in the preceding pages, the form instruction section is more detailed, though it also is much like any form instruction in any martial arts manual. There are two parts. Part one begins with the state of non-polarity—the state of relaxed emptiness before the practitioner commences the form. From there, it goes into the drills that embody the Five Elements: chopping, crashing, drilling, blasting, and crossing. Part one finishes with a form that combines all five drills into a unified whole.

Part two contains the forms for Xingyi's other notable stable of movements: the Twelve Animals. These are: Dragon, Tiger, Monkey, Horse, Alligator, Rooster, Hawk, Swallow, Snake, Kestral, Eagle, and Bear. As with part one, part two ends with a combined form. The verbal descriptions in both part one and part two are accompanied by photos of a relatively young Sun, sans beard. A single photo depicts each movement.

The book winds up with a sparring section showing how Xingyi operates against an opponent. The illustrations here are in an older-style of Chinese drawing. This section concludes the book.

There is a lot of form work displayed in this book, and since Xingyi is such a basic linear art, it might be a simple task to learn it from these pages. But maybe more important is the book's value as a resource for Xingyi practitioners wishing to get as close to the art's roots as possible. The major drawback is the paucity of background, philosophy, and principles of the art.

A Study of Bagua Boxing

Sun's second book, *A Study of Bagua Boxing*, is easily one of his best. Like the others, it is a basic manual containing Bagua's background, philosophy, methodology, and so forth, before moving on to the instruction section. This is followed by several chapters that are more philosophical and spiritual in content. But much of the material throughout, while succinct, has more depth than is usual for a book of this type—though that proclivity has somewhat changed for the better over the years.

The book opens with prefaces by Chen Weiming and Wu Xinggu, both of whom wrote similar prefaces to Sun's *A Study of Taiji Boxing* (below). But there is a passage of note in Chen's preface in which Sun gives his rationale for publishing books and teaching many students. (Material in brackets is added by translator Brennan.):

> He said to me, "No matter how detailed and comprehensively I explain things, even if I am talking to those who seem capable of understanding, only one or two out of a hundred get it, and so I worry these arts will cease to be passed down." [In other words, it's a numbers game. The more people he shares with, the larger will be that population of the understanding few.]

This sort of statement is the kind made by a true master who is concerned about the vitality and longevity of the arts he practices. The truth these days is that the martial arts have never been so vital. Most action movies and TV shows display a plethora of styles, and where there were once but a few handfuls of martial arts actors, there are now hundreds—maybe thousands. And while the purist might argue that cinematic martials arts aren't really martial arts, I might argue otherwise. Many of these actors can clearly kick butt and some have a deep, perhaps profound, understanding of the martial arts. My point is that the martial arts are thriving at all levels worldwide.

But back to our topic. Sun's own preface comes next. It is short but manages to lay out the importance of the *I Ching* (*Book of Changes*) to Bagua and to skim the history of the art.

Next comes a section titled, "General Comments," to which translator Brennan adds: "Much of the text here is reused from Sun's Xingyi manual." It's easy to see how Sun might have done that by substituting "Bagua" for "Xingyi" in the text since most of the material here is very generic, though centered on the internal as opposed to the external martial arts. So it's all pretty basic stuff, but it's the kind of stuff that bears frequent repeating. Some of the points, however, are concerned only with Bagua. For example:

> This boxing art is not only convenient for solo practice, but for group practice as well. A single circle can accommodate up to three or even five people. Dozens of people, even hundreds or more can practice together, divided up into many circles.

When I read that, I had a flash of some huge plaza where hundreds of Bagua players occupying scores of interlocking circles move around the circles in an intricate dance, like the gears of cosmic wheels. Every time they use the single- or double-palm change to turn and start the other way, the whole mechanism changes direction instantly and simultaneously. Imagine the energy that would churn up!

Okay, again back to the topic. Chapter one covers the structure of Bagua and why the art is named that. It is, of course, named after the bagua diagram, which depicts the eight trigrams that make up the sixty-four hexagrams of the *I Ching*. Each of the eight trigram consists of three lines that are some combination of either solid (——) or broken (— —), and the total number of pairings of the eight trigrams is sixty-four. The *I Ching* uses these pairings to deliver prognostications based on the energy pattern reflected by the various configurations of the broken and unbroken lines.

Chinese thought concerning the trigrams and hexagrams and their relationship to the reality around us can be seen in many places other than the *I Ching*. Those relationships can get extremely abstruse once one goes into the various possible combinations between the trigrams and their associations with other aspects of reality, such as the five elements (wood, water, metal, fire, air), which also is a notable component of Bagua philosophy. Hence, discussions in Bagua literature can become quite involved and abstract. Thankfully, Sun only takes a toe dip here, not a complete immersion, but it's enough to get a glimpse of the roots of Bagua's deep foundational philosophy.

Chapter two covers the three mistakes that beginners make. All three could have come from any generic internal martial arts manual: Don't use excessive energy (hard or unbalanced energy), don't use awkward effort (muscular force), and don't stick out your chest and lift your belly. These are repeated so often in internal martial arts literature that they could be a mantra, which also means they're good advice.

Chapter three delves into the nine requirements at the beginning of training. I'll just list these, using Sun's own terminology, and let you go to the book itself for more clarity on these ideas:

1) Sinking
2) Hollowing
3) Lifting
4) Pressing
5) Wrapping
6) Loosening
7) Hanging
8) Shrinking
9) Clearly distinguishing between lifting, drilling, dropping, and overturning

Most of these are self-explanatory or are already familiar to internal stylists, but the last is fairly interesting and shows how Sun can pack a lot of information into a small space.

> As for "lifting, drilling, dropping, and overturning": lifting is drilling and dropping is overturning. Lifting is horizontal and dropping is vertical. Lifting and drilling are threading. Dropping and overturning are striking. But when lifting is also striking, dropping is still striking. Strike with lifting and dropping, like the wheels of machinery spinning continuously.

There go those whirling cosmic wheels again, but probably that's only natural for an art that practices by walking a circle.

After defining these nine requirements, Sun goes a little more deeply into how the energy flows around the circle and through the various trigrams, altering in character and function as it does. There's some intricate reasoning here that I won't go into, but again, one passage begs to be noted:

Although the arts of Xingyi and Bagua are divided into associations with the square circle and the round circle, their theory is simply to restrain your power while moving, causing your energy to consolidate and return to your elixir field.

At the time he wrote this, Sun had yet to learn Taiji, but if he had, no doubt he'd have added it to his description.

Next comes a chapter covering Bagua boxing's four virtues, eight abilities, and four basic situations. Again, I'll simply list and leave it to you to read Sun's own brief but pithy explications. The four virtues are:

1) Going along
2) Going against
3) Harmoniousness
4) Transformation

The eight abilities are:

1) Parrying
2) Blocking
3) Checking
4) Covering
5) Pushing
6) Propping
7) Leading
8) Guiding

The four basic situations are:

1) Lifting
2) Drilling
3) Dropping
4) Overturning

You will notice that the theme of the square and the octagon are continued here, and Sun spends some time linking different aspects of all of these virtues, abilities, situations, and movements via the bagua diagram.

Chapter five distinguishes left and right circle walking, and the next four chapters delve into the postures known as non-polarity and grand polarity, which are the states of non-movement then internal preparation for movement—essentially standing there, centering and relaxing oneself, then energizing your body to prepare for movement. Taijiquanists utilize the same methodology in Preparation to Open Taiji.

Then it's time for the form instruction section. Sun breaks the form into easy-to-digest sections, each of which is relatively short in terms of number of movements. Each section links to the one before it, and each is prefaced with information about the performance, meaning, and application of the movements in the section. Warnings also are included. When writing about a particular technique, for example, Sun says:

> A moment of two-fingered pressure can cause sudden death. This method can be understood but must not be deliberately used.

But promises of better things also are there:

> When the energy in your elixir field is sufficient, then your Daoist mind will be born. Once your Daoist mind is born, passive fire in your heart will be dispelled, and you will be without dizziness and blurry vision.

The form instruction section, of course, occupies most of the book, and a careless reader might not realize that buried beneath all of that, at the back of the book, rests a treasure. In five brief chapters, Sun delivers some of the most interesting material of any of his writings. Here, he goes into some depth regarding internal energy and its genesis and development through deliberate acquisition, and he further explicates the bagua diagram and its relationship to the art and reality. Other topics include "the attributes of active fire and passive compliance in Bagua," "the attributes of refining spirit and returning to emptiness in Bagua," and, finally, "on time and place in Bagua's training for spiritual transformation." The material in these five chapters is meaningful and important for any internal martial artist, regardless of style, making this one of Sun's best and most important books.

A Study of Bagua Sword

Sun Lutang might have been a master of the internal martial arts, but this book does not contain any outstanding insights. Instead, it is a standard-issue introduction to and instruction for Bagua sword. As such, it is generally no better or worse than most such manuals, except for the fact that it is by Sun Lutang, who not only was closer to the genesis of Bagua than most other writers on the subject but also was closer to the heart of the art than just about anybody else.

The book opens with a preface by Wu Xingu, which discusses a couple of elements of Bagua in general terms. Following that, Sun presents his own preface, which is brief enough since he states that the origins of Bagua sword are unknown but that it was disseminated in Beijing by Dong Haichuan. Sun's own teacher, Cheng Tinghua, was Dong's disciple. The preface goes on to elaborate the eight-trigram theory that dominates Bagua philosophy. He finishes, however, by stating that Bagua sword ought to be called Taiji sword because of its adherence to polarities.

Sun then goes on to discuss the idea that external appearances are of much less consequence than is imbuing one's sword with vital energy. He then goes into the dynamics of Bagua circle walking. His descriptions are very detailed, and toward the end of this section, they take into account the sword's relationship to the footwork.

A discussion of hand positions comes next, and those for each hand are detailed—and I do mean in detail. What Sun calls the "eight essential terms in sword practice" are listed, each with a brief description, and this is followed by a chapter titled: "The Distinction in Bagua Sword of Left and Right Circle Walking and Left and Right Sword or Hand Threading." A couple of sections on non-polarity and grand polarity postures wind up the introductory material. Non-polarity is essentially wuwei, or the state of non-action, and the posture is the same as Taiji's beginning posture before commencement of the form. Grand polarity, as noted above, is the moment in which the flow of internal energy begins but before it manifests.

The form instruction section comes next and occupies almost all of the remainder of the book. As with most such instruction sections, this one has explanatory text accompanied by a single photo of Sun performing the posture. The form is broken into eight subforms, each named for one of Bagua's eight trigrams, and while the single photo accompanying each individual movement isn't really adequate, the explanations are very detailed. This probably would be valuable material for any Bagua sword enthusiast.

The next chapter covers Bagua sword's ten basic actions, which are explained briefly in practical combat terms: Your opponent does that, you do this. The final chapter is on the essentials of Bagua sword's unfixed practice, or, mixing up and embellishing the basic actions to make your sword technique flexible and unpredictable.

All-in-all, this is probably one of the best Bagua sword manuals out there, though I certainly don't have more than a cursory knowledge of others that might sit on the shelves of the ultimate martial arts library. Among those is another translation of this same book done by Franklin Fick, which is not covered in this series.

A Study of Taiji Boxing

Amazon.com shows a dozen or so books devoted to Sun Style Taiji, some by Sun Lutang, some by or in cooperation with his daughter, Sun Jianyun. What we consider here is the original Sun Style manual, authored by the founder himself. I'll note here that there is at least one other translation of this same book done by notable martial artist Tim Cartmell, but I have not compared the two versions.

Sun Lutang already was an acknowledged master of Bagua and Xingyi when he learned Wu/Hao Style from Hao Wei-chen, beginning in 1911. He later was invited by Yang Shaohou, Yang Chenfu, and Wu Chienchuan to teach at the Beijing Physical Education Research Institute. During his years there, Yang, Wu, and Sun Styles all underwent significant development.[5] Because Sun was developed out of of Wu/Hao, it could be said that all the styles that were direct offshoots of Chen Style were represented at the institute. Undoubtedly there would have been a co-mingling of efforts and understandings among these significant masters.

A Study of Taiji Boxing opens with a couple of prefaces by invitees—Chen Weiming and Wu Xingu—and both are standard fare for books of this sort. The author's preface, however, which comes next, puts considerable more meat on the bones. It begins with a mystical description of the creation of the universe and the separation of the primordial energies into yin and yang. This in turn morphs into the world of form—the ten thousand things. Sun quickly moves on to the conventional story of Damo/Bodhidharma traveling to and residing at the Shaolin Temple and teaching the monks the rudiments of chi kung and kung fu.

Sun then discusses several Taiji principles, such as the use of acquired postures, but not of acquired strength:

> In every movement and stillness, it is entirely natural, never emphasizing animal vigor, for its purpose is to transform energy into spirit.

There follows a somewhat detailed explanation of how Taiji moves from "the single principle to the nine palaces, then returns to the single principle." Each of the "nine palaces" is defined, but I'll leave that to Sun. I will, though, give an extended quote that I think is important, especially given the personal expertise of the author:

> I received instruction from Hao, practicing daily for several years, and came to somewhat understand the general principles within the art. I also deeply pondered upon my own experiences from my previous training, and then the three arts of Xingyi Boxing, Bagua Boxing, and Taiji Boxing merged to become a single essence. This single essence is yet separated into the three distinct systems. The postures of the three systems are different, but their principles are the same.

Next, the story of Zhang (Chang) Sanfeng's development of Taiji and its dispersal via Wang Zongue (Tsung-yueh) is briefly recounted, and after that, Sun describes, also briefly, his own journey through the internal martial arts.

The following chapter, "The Name 'Taiji Boxing'", discusses how the art conforms—physically, mentally, and spiritually—to the concept of the interplay of yin and yang, as embodied in the taijitu, or the tai chi symbol. Topics touched on are flow, expansion and contraction, continuousness, and interchange of energy.

All this material is too brief considering it is from a master who probably had so much more to say. A short chapter that lays out the remainder of the book and another that contains a form list come next, then Sun moves into movement through the form instruction section. This occupies most of the remainder of the book. The textual descriptions are accompanied by one photo per unique movement, which means that toward the end of this section, there are few photos. The photos are murky, which is a reflection of the time when this book first appeared, when photo reproduction techniques and technology were not as developed as they are today.

A chapter on push hands is next, mostly covering tui shou. After that, Sun transcribes the Taiji Classics written by Li Yiyu, which is appropriate considering Li's place in Wu/Hao Style history. Plus, the Classics are always a good reminder of Taiji principles, and can be read profitably time and again. With those, the book ends.

A Study of Taiji Boxing might be distinguished by its author, but it really is a basic martial arts manual that only skims the great depths of the Taiji ocean. Because of its source, it would be essential for Sun Style practitioners, but the information not directly attached to Sun Style can be readily found—often better—in most Taiji books of this sort.

Essays by Sun Lutang

Essays by Sun Lutang is a collection of essays that Sun wrote between 1929 and 1932. All were published in various Chinese martial arts publications of the time. Translator Paul Brennan states at the beginning that these are "important essays," but to my mind, only one contains real substance.

That one is the first: "Discussing Distinctions Between the Internal and External Schools of Martial Arts," written in 1929 but not published until it appeared in the *Yin County Martial Arts Institute 1st Year Commemorative Publication*, 1931. This essay delves into the distinction commonly made among Chinese martial artists between the external/hard/Shaolin martial arts and the internal/soft/Wudang martial arts. In this work, Sun begins with a relatively brief but succinct overview of the commonly held beliefs regarding this sort of categorization, followed by a few paragraphs on his own early approach to the matter.

Seeking further knowledge, he then visited with Song Shirong of Shanxi to learn more on the subject. It was natural for Sun to turn to Song, who was a successor to Li Luoneng, a 19th century popularizer of Xingyi and martial arts brother of Sun's own teacher, Guo Yunshen. Much of the remainder of the essay is Song's take on the external/internal distinction. "Can I say I've obtained the internal power of boxing arts?" he asks Song. "My energy has sunk down and my lower abdomen is hard as a rock." Song's answer is, "Oh, no, no, no. Even though energy might be getting through to your lower abdomen, if it doesn't transform that hardness, it'll eventually just make you feel overworked, and that isn't the highest level."

It quickly becomes clear that, for Song, the distinction between the external and internal has less to do with history (Shaolin vs Wudang) or method (hard vs soft), but more to do with breathing that leads to a relaxed inner harmony. He says:

> If this is not clear, then even if you practice until you are as agile as a fluttering bird or strong enough to lift a ton, you will be no more than a brash oaf and always will be of the external school. If instead you train to the point of centered harmoniousness...then even if you are a mass of muscle, you can be considered one of the internal school.

Song's pithy words helped Sun discover for himself "that the way of boxing arts is the way of Nature, and that the way of Nature is the way of mankind."

I have only skimmed the surface of this essay in this review, but it is a strong work of value to any martial artist, though perhaps mostly for those of the internal school, to help guide them along the path of least resistance.

The collection's second essay is "Some Things I Have Been Told About Martial Arts," published in the *Jiangsu Martial Arts Institute Annual* in 1929. Sun begins this essay with his own dabbling in various styles as a youth and young man, discovering "that the way of the boxing arts is all-encompassing, embodying everything with nothing left out." The implication of this statement is that his broad introduction to the Chinese martial arts led him to become master of several internal styles and resulted in his syncretic Sun Style Taiji.

Sun then relates portions of conversations he later had with several individuals who seemed to advance Sun's syncretic approach. The first is Gao Daofu, a master calligrapher who was one of Sun's students. In this conversation, Gao likens the martial arts to calligraphy, noting not just that both the martial artist and the calligrapher must exhibit a fluidity free from tension, but that there often are abstract structural similarities. As an example, he likens the five elements of Xingyi to the five strokes used in calligraphy. An interesting aspect here is Sun's unspoken presumption that students can teach the teacher, and that each person can bring to his art—martial or fine—individual viewpoints that can advance his or her understanding of any sort of human endeavor.

The second conversation is with Li Jinglin, a military supervisor and founder of the Warrior's Society. According to Sun, Li was an exquisite Taiji swordsman who concluded that sword art theory "touches upon everything, thereby connecting it to all other systems." Indeed, even his military experiences in strategy and battlefield tactics had an effect on his sword theory.

The third conversation is with another swordsman, Zhuang Sijian, who was a clerk in the Records Bureau. "What Li practices," Zhuang told Sun, "is Taiji Sword, and what I practice is Bagua Sword. Although the two styles are different, their methods of application are fifty or sixty percent the same, and they share the same names of the different grip positions." Sun tells Zhuang that "the principles of the boxing arts and sword arts roughly amount to three:

1) Above and below coordinate with each other.

2) Neither reaching nor separating, neither coming away nor crashing in, neither under-involved nor over-involved.
3) The boxing is without boxing. The intention is without intention.

In response, Zhuang agrees, taking us full circle back to calligraphy: "This actually is the same as in the rules, spirit, structure, transitioning, and manner of calligraphy."

The third essay in the collection is "My Opinions on the Origins of Chinese Martial Arts," originally published in the *Collection of Articles from the Zhejiang Martial Arts and Recreation Conference, 1930*. In this short work, Sun lays out his version of Chinese martial arts history, beginning with pre-historic Chinese emulating animal movements. He then very briefly covers the Yellow Emperor's contributions to martial arts development and the following development of the arts through several dynasties.

The legendary Damo/Bodhidharma traveling to the Shaolin Temple makes an appearance, as does Taiji's legendary creator, Chang Sanfeng, and this segues quickly to mere mentions of several styles subsequently developed from Shaolin and Wudang martial arts. The author concludes with this statement:

> Narrow-mindedness toward other styles leads to snobbery, and so I fervently hope that throughout the nation it is the broadminded masters who are doing the teaching.

Unfortunately, that eventuality seems unlikely, at least in the world in which we presently live.

This essay is easily the weakest and most facile in the collection. Sun's history is too terse to deliver much information, and the information it does deliver relies on the standard semi-mythic take on Chinese martial arts development. Better—and more accurate—histories can be found in many other sources.

The final essay is, "A Detailed Look at the Theories of Xingyi, Bagua, and Taiji," published in a 1932 issue of *Martial Arts Weekly*. Sun opens the essay by distinguishing three broad categories of Chinese martial arts: Shaolin, Wudang, and Emei. The first two are probably familiar to most practitioners of the Chinese martial arts, but the third is more obscure. Emei, or more properly:

Emeiquan, is a group of Chinese martial arts from Mount Emei in Sichuan Province.... It is known for its swiftness and flexibility...and is known for its animal-based fighting methods.[6]

In saying this, I've told you more about Emeiquan than Sun does in this fairly long essay. Instead, Sun focuses on the three major internal arts of Xingyi, Bagua, and Taiji, and there is some pithy information here for internal martial artists of each school. Each art is treated to about a page of text that lays out the principles and tenets of the art: Xingyi's five core movements and twelve animal imitations, Bagua's adherence to the sixty-four hexagrams of the *I Ching*, and Taiji's centered harmoniousness. He concludes, "By analogy, Xingyi is the ground, Bagua is the sky, and Taiji is mankind." And in keeping with Sun's syncretic approach to the internal martial arts, he then states, "The three substances of sky, ground, and mankind are merged into a single whole, mixed into a union with no meaningful distinctions."

Authentic Explanations of Martial Arts Concepts

This book cannot be properly said to be "by" Sun Lutang, but rather he serves as compiler and editor of statements and concepts elucidated by other masters of the Chinese martial arts, most of whom Sun studied under or with.

It begins with a preface by Chen Weiming, himself a significant master and disseminator of Yang Style Taiji and author on the art. Next is a preface by Wu Xingu, about whom I know nothing. Both prefaces speak to Sun's background and expertise. These are followed by a preface by the author in which he talks in general terms about the three major Chinese internal martial arts systems—Xingyi, Bagua, and Taiji—which he is famous for synthesizing into a comprehensive style.

Then it's on to the main substance of the book, which consists of three major sections. The first section contains brief biographies of the masters whose teachings he distills in the second section. The third section contains a chapter on compiling highlights from

Xingyi, and that is followed by a chapter relating Sun's personal experiences of practicing the three systems and essential concepts within them. The major emphasis in the book is on Xingyi, perhaps because that is the system Sun studied longest—first love, and all that. There are fourteen bios of Xingyi masters, two of Bagua masters, and three of Taiji masters. The bios are generally only a paragraph or two, though some occupy a full page. Some of these masters are significant enough to have somewhat longer online bios in sources such as *Wikipedia*, but others are more obscure to Western readers, so their inclusion here is valuable.

The breakdown in the chapters distilling the teachings of these masters has a similar spread, with teachings by fourteen Xingyi masters, only one Bagua master, and two Taiji masters. This section contains the real meat of the book as the various masters relay, though Sun, good, solid information. But don't think that because the lion's share of the pages are devoted to Xingyi that Bagua and Taiji exponents won't find much value here. Although some of the statements and concepts are system-specific, most of the information is pan-system—that is, applicable to any internal system. As for the concepts that are system-specific, they provide valuable insights into the workings of that system.

The penultimate chapter containing highlights from Xingyi manuals contains information similar to that divulged in the preceding chapters, while the final chapter, relaying Sun's personal experiences, is important for the insights this historically significant master imparts. In it, he discusses how the body reacts to internal martial arts training, internal energy, the meditative quality of emptiness inherent in these arts, breathing, and elixerism. He finishes the chapter with a section on unconscious awareness developed by practicing emptiness and joining with the Way.

Conclusion

With *The Complete Works of Sun Lutang*, Paul Brennan has made a significant contribution to English-language martial arts literature. His translations are professional-grade, using clear and precise phrasings to relay the knowledge contained in these books in a highly readable format.

Also interesting are the photos of Sun on the title pages of several of the books—scans courtesy of the translator. Photos of Sun in books and on the web typically are shots of him as an older or old man, with his trademark long whiskers and serious demeanor. (As in the shot of him at the beginning of this review.) That's the case with most of the photos in these books, but a couple show him as a younger man. The earlier of the two, in *A Study of Bagua Boxing*, depicts a young Sun in full-dress uniform as a Junior Field Officer at the Presidential Palace, for which he served as a captain in "Scholar Tiger" section. In this photos, he has no facial hair. The second shows a more mature Sun in a dark jacket with a high collar and sporting a mustache.

In many ways, Sun's most important legacy is not the schools that have built up since his death around his various martial arts. It is, instead, the idea that if you understand and can embody one of the internal martial arts, then in many ways and to one degree or another, you can understand and embody them all. Everything else is style of movement training and catalogs of martial technique. The true essence is not the martial but the art, for that is transmitted via the way the body is trained to move. The more sophisticated and efficient the movement, the more effective the martial art, not only for self-defense/fighting and health/well-being, but for producing satisfying emotional and philosophical content.

Sun Lutang was a master of three internal martial arts, which meant that he had learned to deeply embody each style as an individual art. But his greatest achievement was in combining all three as one. For him, free and intentional multidimensional movement was real, and he was happy to share with others the possibilities inherent in that fact as well as the methods one could use to achieve similar results.

Notes
1 "Sun Lutang," *Wikipedia* (https://en.wikipedia.org/wiki/Sun_Lutang
2 "Aikido." *Wikipedia*, https://en.wikipedia.org/wiki/Aikido
3. "Shotokan." *Wikipedia*, https://en.wikipedia.org/wiki/Shotokan

4. "History of Wing Chun." *Wikipedia*, https://en.wikipedia.org/wiki/History_of_Wing_Chun

5. "Sun Lutang." *Wikipedia*, https://en.wikipedia.org/wiki/Sun_Lutang

6 "Emeiquan." *Wikipedia*, https://en.wikipedia.org/wiki/Emeiquan

Links

International Sun Style Tai Chi Association: http://www.suntaichi.com/news.html

Combat Techniques of Taiji, Xingyi, and Bagua
Principles and Practices of Internal Martial Arts

By Lu Shengli
(Blue Snake Books, 2006, 372 pages)

Combat Techniques of Taiji, Xingyi, and Bagua by Lu Shengli is a handsome book filled with excellent and thorough information delivered in clear, measured language. It might well have been subtitled, "A Family Portrait," since the three arts it discusses are closely related in philosophy and methodology if not specific techniques. Lu learned the three arts from several masters, most significantly Wang Peisheng. (See Volume VI of this series for a review of Wang's Taiji book.) His training was long, arduous, and deep, lending his book an air not just of competence, but of intelligent contemplation.

The book begins with two long forewords, one by translator and editor Zhang Yun, and the second by one of Lu's students, Strider Clark. Unlike many such forwards, which contain only rote praise, these also help characterize the personality, mindset, and martial expertise of the author. Lu's preface comes next, and in it, he describes who he is, how he came to the martial arts, and his general philosophy on them. What he says sounds pretty good to me.

Chapter one covers the basic principles of the internal martial arts. The distinctions between Neijia Quan (internal martial arts)

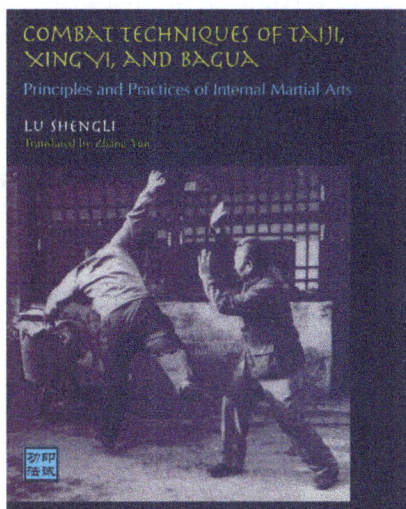

and Waijia Quan (external martial arts) is made, but Lu is quick to point out that the distinctions are not hard-and-fast lines but are somewhat flexible. While some arts (Taiji, Bagua, and Xingyi) are primarily internal, and Shaolin-style arts are primarily external, others, such as Baji Quan, Tongbei Quan, and Sanhuang Paochui Quan are mixtures of internal and external.

Following this thoughtful delineation that takes in many aspects and characteristics of both these two basic schools of martial arts, Lu goes into the development of the Chinese martial arts in general, saying that external styles came first, with internal styles later providing an alternative way of combat. His information is detailed and seems well researched, and I'm inclined to accept much of his take on Chinese martial history. This is especially true when he lays out various alternative histories of the development of these arts, from the wildest tall tales to the most rational of views on the topic, almost always landing on the side of the latter. But that doesn't mean he ignores the wild histories of Taiji, Bagua, and Xingyi—or even disparages them—since he knows that, first, they are important parts of martial arts lore; second, they are entertaining; and third, they sometimes relay something of value regarding the principles and methodology of the martial arts they concern.

The next section looks in greater detail at the main differences between Waijia and Neijia, which entails discussions of Buddhism and Taoism, the human capacity to increase or change natural ability, training methods (outside to inside and inside to outside), external and internal jin, and fighting strategies.

Next come three sections, one each on Xingyi, Taiji, and Bagua, in that order, from eldest to youngest—at least in terms of verifiable historicity. Each of these sections has a similar structure. First is a subsection on history and lineage, how the martial art developed into different styles, the differences between them, and notable practitioners. In relating the histories of each art, the author not only names the lineages and major branches, but covers in some detail the progressive etymology of each style's name(s). Even better, he peppers the narrative with tall tales, colorful anecdotes, and character studies of major practitioners, and he does his best to distinguish between fact, informed supposition, and fiction. This is followed by a subsection on the principles and features of the art, including philosophy and precepts, and after that comes a subsection on training methods. Lu also gives somewhat lesser space and detail to Tongbei Quan and Baji Quan.

It is intriguing to read the various versions of the development of a martial art, even of those one does not practice, and I found Lu's sections on Xingyi and Bagua highly detailed and very worthwhile. But being a Taiji guy, I was most interested in his take on the history of that art. It is a convoluted journey, covering what he calls the five legendary forms of Taiji, only the last of which begins with Chang Sanfeng. It is known that internal styles embodying the same principles as Taiji existed for some time prior to the art's historical beginnings with the Chen family, and Lu lends his knowledge of Taiji history to flesh in that shadowy genesis and meandering development. It should be noted that his tacit acceptance of the five strands of Taiji development is not isolated to Lu, but appears in several other histories of Taiji reviewed in this series. The implications of this multiplicity are worth serious consideration. (See the Appendix for a list of books reviewed in this series that deal with alternate histories if Taiji's inception and development.)

The history of Taiji's modern era begins with Yang Luchan learning Taiji from the Chen family. Lu delivers a far more detailed accounts of Yang's association with the Chens than is usually seen. In most versions, Yang finagles his way into the Chen family and learns Taiji while employed by them. In Lu's version, Yang was sold as a slave to the Chens by his uncle and remained their indentured servant for much of his life until finally given his freedom, by which time he'd become excellent at Taiji.

Fundamentals of basic internal martial arts movements and applications are the subjects of the next chapter. Lu does not break these down by specific art, for his intent here is not to continue the existence of the three arts as separate and independent (the already-strong link between Xingyi and Bagua notwithstanding), but to blend them, much as Sun Lutang had done previously, into a single coherent art that embodies and melds the best aspects of the three. Lu's composite form consists of sixteen postures, and it is designed to emphasize combat skills.

So, instead of relying on descriptions of form movements, he breaks things down into individual skills clustered by body part: hand, elbow, shoulder, hip, knee, foot, head, and trunk. Each section contains multiple possibilities for attack or defense, and as might be expected, the section on the use of the hand is the longest and contains the most possibilities. This is all excellent material for internal martial artists of any style and might even add to your repertoire.

A section on stepping comes next, all based on Taiji's five named stances—forward, backward, left, right, and central equilibrium—but Lu adds a few variations on these themes to improve their utility.

Basic kung fu training occupies the next chapter at eighty pages. Adhering to the real meaning of "kung fu"—excellence achieved through effort over time—Lu advances the reader through an arduous and involved set of strengthening and conditioning exercises that have as their foundation Pile Standing (Standing Post). Following this are numerous exercises designed to help the practitioner improve and strengthen the flow of internal energy and are like moving chi kungs. Many philosophical ideas, principles, and precepts are examined here, often in great detail. This stuff would be difficult to practice, but it probably would be worth it if you intend to reach the higher levels of one or more of the internal martial arts. If you're inclined to take it up, I advise you to start at a relatively young age. Some of this is not for oldsters.

In the next chapter, Lu introduces his sixteen-posture form, which he says, "is designed to help middle-level practitioners understand and master the fighting principles and skills of the internal martial arts." This is a pretty standard form instruction, the main difference being the thoroughness and detail of its explanations, each of which includes potential applications. Adequate photos depict each movement and its applications.

The final chapter discusses the practice of applications in tactical terms, focusing on specific application training, assessing the opponent, finding the proper distance, determining timing and direction, moving in various directions, protecting your body, and practicing applications. "Are you ready for fighting?" asks the title of the final section, and Lu answers the question in no-nonsense terms.

Combat Techniques of Taiji, Xingyi, and Bagua is an excellent book powered by deep understanding and conveyed in a simple, straightforward writing style that clearly and concisely delivers the facts and the author's reasonings. While the the superbly detailed information contained and the considerate tenor of the text are undoubtedly Lu's, we should also give credit to the two translators/editors—

Zhang Yun and Susan Darley—for some of the book's helpful structure and excellent English-language version.

The book really has only two detriments—and both are serious. First, it lacks an index. This is a lot of book to try to thumb through to find something specific, which you might want to do considering the quality of the author's knowledge and expertise. And second, the author utilizes a large number of Chinese terms but most often fails to define what they are in English. This is where a comprehensive glossary would be invaluable. Right before that index.

Otherwise, beginners and mid-level practitioners should get a great deal of solid information, no matter which of these arts they practice. Highly recommended.

The Power of the Internal Martial Arts
Combat and Energy Secrets of Ba Gua, Tai Chi, and Hsing-I

by Bruce Frantzis
(Blue Snake Books, 2008, 226 pages)

Martial arts are like containers. The practitioner spends time learning to create a container—the martial art form—and then proceeds to fill the container with content—chi and physiological and martial knowledge and skill. Sometimes the containers (forms) are faulty or misshapen, sometimes they are well formed but remain empty or are only partially filled. Shallow martial knowledge will be evident in these types of forms, and while their practitioners might mimic the true art they purport to represent, their efforts generally fall short of insight and validity, much less mastery. Martial arts books are no different. Each is a container filled with some relative martial knowledge, whether excellent, mediocre, or somewhere between.

At the excellent end of the spectrum lies Bruce Frantzis' *The Power of the Internal Martial Arts*. Part of the reason the book is so good is that Frantzis was an early traveler to Japan, China, India, and elsewhere during his decades-long research into the martial arts. The book is filled with his recollections of the many masters he studied with, but it is perhaps useful to recount a succinct bio up front to give the reader an idea of Frantzis' background. To make sure I'm

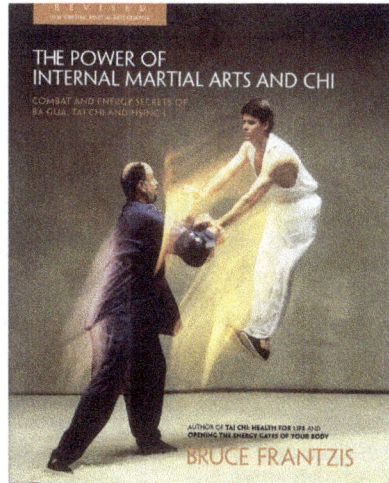

unbiased here, the following bio is pulled directly from the *Wikipedia* page on him, though *that* might be biased:

Bruce Kumar Frantzis (born April 1949) is a Taoist educator who studied Taoism in China. Beginning as a young karate champion, he engaged in a multi-decade journey leading him throughout Asia and the Eastern energetic traditions. Choosing to forgo an ivy league education in favor of pursuing Japanese martial arts at their original source, he moved to Japan to attend Sophia University at the age of eighteen. There, he obtained multiple black belts and trained with Aikido's founder Morihei Ueshiba. He soon branched out to Taiwan and China and studied in increasing depth under internal martial arts masters.

In 1973, attempting to locate the original source of meditation, Bruce traveled to India where he underwent rigorous daily training in Pranayama, Hatha yoga, Raja yoga, and Tantra with many gurus, experiencing what in the East is known as "Kundalini Shakti".

Returning to China in the mid 1970s, he became the first Westerner to be given insider access to the closely guarded Taoist Fire tradition (unverified tradition) and its priesthood. After completing seven years of training he became priest in the Fire tradition. Then by a fortunate set of events, Bruce was accepted as the direct disciple of one of the few remaining stewards of the Water tradition (unverified tradition), the Taoist Immortal (Fully Realized Person) Liu Hung-Chieh. Through Liu Hung-Chieh, he was introduced to Jiang Jia Hua the vice president of the All-China Scientific Qigong Association. This connection gave Bruce access to Chinese cancer clinics where he completed his training as a medical qigong doctor.

Bruce inherited the Taoist Water Tradition lineages shortly before Liu Hung-Chieh's passing in 1986. On his teacher's wishes, he has spent the last 25 years imparting the healing, meditative and martial aspects of Taoism to the West. He primarily teaches the Energy Art Qigong System, Wu style tai chi, ba gua, Taoist Yoga and Taoist Meditation. He has authored numerous works (including *The Power of the Internal*

Martial Arts and Chi, Tao of Letting Go, Dragon and Tiger Medical Qigong, and *Opening the Energy Gates of Your Body*) on Taoist energetic practices and taught over 20,000 students many of whom have gone on to become active certified instructors.[1]

This entry sounds like it was pulled from an advertising brochure, but suffice it to say that Frantzis knows whereof he speaks, and in this book, he speaks volumes about the internal martial arts of Bagua, Taiji, and Xingyi. I'm reviewing here the revised edition (2007), which adds a lengthy section on the spiritual aspects of the internal martial arts to the original edition (1998). I first became aware of Bruce Frantzis in the 1980s through a spate of articles he wrote for *Tai Chi Magazine.* I've also reviewed two of his other books in this series: *The Big Book of Tai Chi: Build Health Fast in Slow Motion* (in Volume V) and *The Chi Revolution: Harness the Power of Your Life Force* (in Volume II).

The Power of the Internal Martial Arts is impressive from the outset. While not being encyclopedic, it manages to cover the three arts in question in significant detail and depth, from their historical origins to their functionality to their strengths and weaknesses. Telegraphing the book's weight, the "Contents" alone occupy eleven pages. In fact, this lengthy book is so packed with information that I'm going to have to gloss through the contents.

The book opens with more prefatory material than you can shake a stick at, including an author's acknowledgements, a forward by Jess O'Brien, a preface by Lee Burkins, sections on the individuals and internal martial arts schools mentioned in the book, a prologue, sections on spiritual malaise, the characteristics of chi masters as teachers, and fa jin. *Then* comes the author's introduction.

Finally, it's on to chapter one, titled "Animal, Human, and Spiritual: Three Approaches to Martial Arts." Here, Frantzis discusses these three approaches, defines the "art" of internal martial arts, and advises the practitioner to train sensibly.

Chapter two—"A Continuum: The External and Internal Martial Arts of China"—defines the parameters of the internal martial arts. Subjects covered are the various types of martial arts and their traditions, the relative quality of the various martial arts, a definition of fighting applications, living and dead forms, and the focus of external martial arts, such as power and strength, speed, endurance, and reflexes. Then it turns to the focus of the internal martial arts—chi—and the reasons that Frantzis emphasizes Bagua in the book. Also touched on are Iron Shirt chi kung and weapons training.

The next chapter looks at the similarities and differences between Taiji, Xingyi, and Bagua and begins with a brief discussion of the five characteristics of internal martial arts. Developing martial power with chi is next on the agenda, focusing mainly on Frantzis' 16-Part Nei Gung Internal Power System. Included is a useful section on what Frantzis calls the "dissolving process," which is a method of releasing blockages of chi. This leads into a section on the stages of feeling the "I" (intention), "Hsin" (heart–mind), and chi and the way the three move. The principal differences and similarities of Taiji, Bagua, and Xingyi are presented next, including footwork and the utilization of the waist and hands, studying the three arts for fighting, basic power training, and the importance of standing practice (Standing Post) for the long-term development of internal power.

The chapter then covers to Bagua's eight stages of practice for developing fighting skills. After delineating the parameters of each stage, Frantzis turns to internal fighting techniques, encompassing a large number of strikes, chin na, throws, kicking, fighting angles, sparring, and fa jin. The next section discusses the martial qualities of small-, medium-, and large-frame methods of movement of Taiji, Xingyi, and Bagua.

Each of the next three chapters focuses in a similar fashion on one of the arts, beginning with Taiji. Matters discussed are Taiji as a martial art, the eight basic martial principles of Taiji, including their overt and covert manifestations. Frantzis then suggests four progressive stages for learning Taiji as a martial art and discusses long and short forms, left- and right-hand forms, push hands, sparring, and fighting. Chapter five does similar justice to Xingyi, and includes a history of the art as well as the training practices, martial techniques, and tools of Xingyi. Chapter six does the same for Bagua.

The nature of speed in all styles of martial arts is the subject of chapter seven. Here, Frantzis breaks speed into four types that he discusses at some length: speed from point A to point B, speed at touch, speed under differing conditions, and speed in relation to power. Included are what the author calls the "fast/slow paradox" of the internal martial arts, qualities in common among the three, and specialized strategies.

The health aspects of the martial arts comes next, beginning with the internal martial arts as energy-healing systems. Some of the subjects discussed are the difference between health and fitness, self-defense vs health benefits, chi kung, repairing agitated chi, healing, aging, and mental health.

"The Tao of Spiritual Martial Arts: A Bridge to Taoist Meditation" is the title of the final chapter, and here Frantzis delves into what a spiritual martial art is and how daunting the spiritual journey can be, for it requires the practitioner to suffer physical, mental, emotional, and spiritual trials in order to heal the individual as well as advance him or her along the road to spiritual enlightenment. As Frantzis points out, this journey is not for the faint-hearted. Perhaps, but from what I can tell, it is a journey we all must take, whether we like it or not, in this lifetime or another.

Seven appendices and an index finish the book, and most of these are interesting in their own right. Subjects are the history of Taiji and characteristics of the various styles, the history of Bagua and its styles, charts of the energy anatomy of the human body, Frantzis's formal lineages and training, Chinese terminology used in the book, and an excellent glossary. The final appendix is composed of vignettes of the subjects that Frantzis teaches, and frankly, this one seems a tad bit self-promotional, almost like they are several pages of non-obvious advertisements. Like the *Wikipedia* article on him.

Scattered throughout the pages are about a dozen profiles of various internal arts masters Frantzis studied with or otherwise encountered, including T. T. Liang, Wang Shu Jin, Cheng Man-ching, Morihei Ueshiba, Yang Shao Jung, and Frantzis' principal teacher, Liu Hung Chieh.

Is this a perfect book on the internal martial arts? No, but can there be such a thing? Some of the information in this book can be found elsewhere, though rarely has this much been compiled under one cover. And despite the voluminous information in this book, there is very little practical instruction. It is an overview of these arts, not the nuts-'n-bolts, though there is enough of the practical to lend depth to the discussions.

On the plus side, the overviews are valuable not just to the practitioners of each of these three arts, but to those who want to know more about the arts they do not practice. And given Frantzis' background, the information is solid and reliable. In addition, he is a good writer, keeping the flow of the text going and illuminating it with illustrative metaphors and nice turns of phrasing.

On the negative side—at least from my personal point of view —Frantzis frequently addresses the raw beginner, but frankly, most of this book will not penetrate a beginner's awareness. In fact, for the beginner, the book might make these arts seem too daunting to attempt. This is a criticism I've had of the two other books by Frantzis that I've read and reviewed. In addition, Frantzis' self-promotion can wear a little thin at times.

But over all, *The Power of the Internal Martial Arts and Chi* is one of the best books on the internal martial arts out there. It's a bit pricey, but you could buy any three cheaper Taiji books for the same amount and not get an equivalent value.

Notes

1 "Bruce Frantzis." *Wikipedia*, https://en.wikipedia.org/wiki/Bruce_Frantzis

PART II

Xingyi & Yiquan

BLANK

Hsing-I
Chinese Mind-Body Boxing

by Robert W. Smith
(Kodansha International, 1974, 112 pages)

The pen of Robert W. Smith produced a number of classic martial arts books. An early American researcher and writer on the martial arts—in particular, the Chinese martial arts—Smith probably wrote more on the subject in English than anyone at the time except Bruce Tegnér or Smith's sometimes co-author, Donn F. Draeger. As is the case with Smith's previous book on Bagua (review below), *Hsing-I* appears to be the first description of the art in English.

Smith opens the book with a chapter on the history of Xingyi, which, like Taiji and Bagua, was developed, it seems, by a mysterious Taoist monk living in remote mountains. Those mysterious Taoist monks sure were a creative lot. Maybe it was all that fresh mountain air and clear spring water. After presenting a chart showing the art's family tree, Smith goes on to delineate the art's two major schools: the Shanshi-Hopei School and the Honan School. A mini-biography of Sun Lutang, who went on to develop Sun Style Taiji, takes up about half of the latter section.

The relationship of Xingyi to Taiji and Bagua is the subject of chapter two. Wrapped up in this is an examination of the stillness/presence inherent in the internal martial arts. Xingyi fundamentals occupy chapter three, and chapter four details the five basic actions

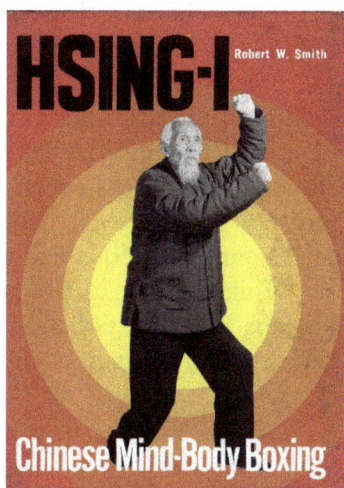

of Xingyi. These are: splitting, crushing, drilling, pounding, and crossing. Each of these are given a thorough explication before Smith shows how to link them together into a single routine. Then comes an application section in which Smith demonstrates several uses for each basic action.

Chapter five is titled, "The Twelve Styles," and it covers the dozen auxiliary movements that have been added to the five basic movements. Chapter six shows the Consecutive Step Yunnan Boxing, which links several movements into a single sequence that once was standard practice by Chinese Nationalist soldiers. Functions follow the form description. Longish chapter seven contains words of Xingyi wisdom from a number of significant masters: Kuo Yunshen, Pai Hsiyuan, Liu Chilan, Sung Shih-jung, Che Ichai, Chang Shute, and many others.

Throughout, there are plenty of photos to illustrate the movements. In the introduction, Smith apologizes for the diversity of the people in the photos, who often are his various teachers and fellow students. I counted seven different individuals in addition to Smith himself. No apology necessary. They all look proficient, and the photos are all adequate at the very least.

While this book will find its primary readership among Xingyi, and perhaps Bagua, exponents, the words of wisdom from the masters in chapter seven contain plenty of substance for Taiji folks, as well.

Selected Subtleties of the Xingyi Boxing Art

By Liu Dianchen
(Originally 1921, *Brennan Translations*, 2012, 104 pages)

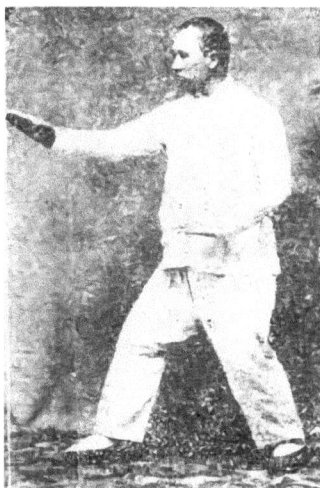

Xingyi, reputedly derived from early spear forms, is a direct and aggressive open-hand internal style that produces explosive power generally delivered at close range. Liu Dianchen, author of *Selected Subtleties of the Xingyi Boxing Art*, was in an excellent position to write a book on it.

Since, Xingyi's roots go back to the dawn of the martial arts in China, its exact origins and early development remain in the realm of mystery, myth, and conjecture. However, if one counts only from the historical beginnings of Xingyi, Ji Longfeng was the first person definitively known to teach the art in historical times. He taught Cao Jiwu, who taught Ma Xueli and Dai Longbang. Each of these last two developed their own distinctive styles, and it is Dai's branch that we will follow. Dai transmitted the art to his clan, and which taught it to Li Luoneng, who taught it to author Liu's father, Liu Qilan. Thus, author Liu enjoyed a position in the direct lineage, and only a few generations removed from the the art's earliest known progenitor.

The book opens with six prefaces, only the last of which is by the author, and only that one contains any real information: on the lineage history of Xingyi. The others are largely throwaways whose authors admit that, while they are familiar with the author, they don't know anything about Xingyi.

Chapter one is on the importance of what the author calls the "Elixir Field," but which most writers on the martial arts refer to as the tantien. One of the purposes of training, Liu says, is to fill the tantien with chi energy that can be wielded as necessary, and he gives a few hints on how to further empower the chi:

1) The insides should be lifted.
2) The three centers should combine (the center of the head top, the center of the soles of the feet, and the centers of the palms).
3) The three intentions should be linked (intentions of mind, energy, and power).
4) The five elements should be smooth.
5) The four antennas should work in unison (tongue, fingers, toes, pores)
6) The mind should be leisurely.
7) The three structure points should align (nose, hands, feet).
8) The eyes should be venomous (eyes should be connected to the energy).

Each of these points is adequately expounded on in one or more paragraphs.

Chapter three covers the movements of muscles in the head, torso, and limbs. A couple of small and definitely inadequate illustrations point out the muscles—if you can actually discern the faint numbers pointing to the various muscles, that is.

Chapter four discusses the Six Unions:

External
    1) Hand with foot
    2) Elbow with knee
    3) Shoulder with hip
Internal
    4) Mind united with intent
    5) Intent united with energy (chi)
    6) Energy united with power

Adhering to these unions help unify the body so that the practitioner can deliver full-body power.

Chapter seven is on the Seven Quicknesses:

1) The eyes should be quick
2) The hands should be quick
3) The feet should be quick
4) The intention should be quick
5) The posture should be quick
6) Advancing and retreating should be quick
7) The whole body should be quick

As with the other numbered lists preceding this one, all the entries are covered by good textual explanations. It's evident by now that the author is enamored of numbered lists to deliver information in an ordered and succinct manner.

The next chapter discusses lifting and dropping, drilling and overturning, and horizontal and vertical. The author states that these terms are apt to challenge the beginner, so he defines each and distinguishes it from the others.

The remainder of the book is devoted to form instruction, first in an open-hand form, then straight sword and spear, which closes the book.

This Xingyi manual would be valuable to practitioners of the art, particularly for the photos of Liu's forms, which predate the modern era. For other readers, there will be less to grasp hold of, although the history sections would be of some interest to the general martial arts historian.

Five Elements Manual

Continuous Boxing Manual

By Li Cunyi
(Originally published c. 1916. *Brennan Translations*, 2017, 39 pages)

This translation from Paul Brennan comprises two short manuals: *Five Elements Manual* and *Continuous Boxing Manual*, both dictated by Li Cunyi, a prominent Xingyi and Bagua stylist. Li was one of the first Xingyi masters to author a book on the art, and his expertise is unquestioned, and his experience is broad and deep. In their *Chinese Martial Arts Training Manuals*, martial arts historians Brian Kennedy and Elizabeth Guo quote Li from his book, *Yue Fe's Intent Boxing*:

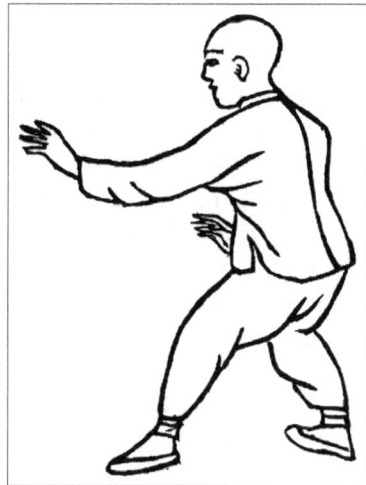

> In order to study martial arts, one must be diligent in two areas. First, one must be willing to travel great distances in order to study with those of higher ability and sincerely request instruction. Second, one must also be diligent in speech, humbling one's self and asking for guidance.[1]

Apparently, Li also was willing to travel far to use his skills to kill people. Kennedy writes:

Li Cun Yi was a prominent Chinese martial arts master of the Xingyi and Bagua systems, but his moral fiber left much to be desired. During the Boxer Rebellion he personally murdered unarmed missionaries and went on to publicly brag about it.[2]

Well, nobody ever said that martial artists aren't as screwed up as everybody else, they're just more dangerous about it. Give a man a weapon, and his next desire is to use it. And Xingyi is a pretty potent weapon: direct, aggressive, powerful and filled with internal energy. And despite the fact that only in Li's generation was the art more widely known and disseminated, it had been around since the dawn of the Chinese martial arts—well, maybe not the dawn, but certainly the early morning.

Five Elements Manual and *Continuous Boxing Manual* are both basic instruction in Xingyi. The former opens with a general introduction that covers Five Element theory, upon which Xingyi is based. Right after that, Li divulges the basic five techniques of crashing, drilling, chopping, blasting, and crossing. You can tell from these names that the style is hard, even if it is classified as internal. Then Li associates each of the techniques in terms of the Five Elements, in which each element destroys another of the elements and is, in turn, destroyed by a third, all the way around the pentagram.

Li next discusses what are called the "Four Antennas":

> The body has blood, muscles, sinews, and bones. The endpoints of these tissues are called "antennas." The antenna of the blood is the hair, the antenna of the muscles is the tongue, the antenna of the sinews is the nails, and the antenna of the bones is the teeth. When the four antennas express power, they can transform you into something unearthly, transmitting to the opponent that he should fear you.

Following that passage are four poems that describe the attributes of each antenna and how each can serve to intimidate an opponent.

Next, Li lists and describes what he calls the "Eight Terms."

Once you have settled into the boxing postures, you are ready for the eight terms. They are all means of storing power and nurturing energy, keeping one who would fight against you from having a way to get started. They are special qualities of the Five Elements.

They are:

1) Three Pressings
2) Three Coverings
3) Three Roundnesses
4) Three Cruelties
5) Three Wrappings
6) Three Lowerings
7) Three Bendings
8) Three Straightenings

You'll have to read the book to get Li's take on each of these.

In keeping with his use of lists to deliver information, Li then gives nine pointers on body alignments:

1) Body
2) Shoulders
3) Forearms
4) Hands
5) Fingers
6) Thighs
7) Feet
8) Tongue
9) Tailbone

Each is briefly described, then it's on to the specific practice of each of the five techniques of crashing, drilling, chopping, blasting, and crossing. Each is treated as a single movement that starts, acts, and finishes, and each concludes with instructions on turning around. Each is accompanied by text, a single simple but basically adequate line drawing, and a crude but effective footwork chart.

After this instruction section, Li discusses a couple of integral aspects of martial arts practice: concentrated practice and long-term practice, pointing out that practicing the martial arts for health is more significant than practicing them for fighting.

> The practice of boxing arts is eighty percent solo practice, twenty percent partner practice. Thus it is said: "Strengthening the body is constant. Defeating opponents is temporary."

Li also encourages the practitioner to focus on a limited number of styles.

> If you are practicing too many techniques," he writes, "you will be neglecting all of them.

As for the idea of long-term practice, Li writes:

> "So deep there is no bottom, so vast there is no horizon." Boxing arts are like this. If you achieve a shallow level you may be able to deal with an opponent, but if you achieve the deepest level, you will be able to deal with any number of them.... A superficial person will look at the contents of the art and feel the the finish line is no better than the starting line, that the long-term achievement is no better than the short-term achievement. However, once your skill has ripened, you will be filled with internal strength.... Mastery comes from two things: humility and perseverance.

The first book closes with variations on each of the five techniques.

Manual for the Continuous Boxing Set comes next, and in it, the five techniques laid out in the previous book are put into a continuous ten-posture form that includes advancing and retreating. Instructions for the form take up the entire book, and each movement has textual instructions and line drawings similar to the ones in the first book but with a twist. In each illustration, there is a figure drawn with dashed lines to indicate the beginning posture and another in solid lines to show the finished posture, with dashed lines on the "floor" to show the movement of the feet.

Xingyi's Five Element theory might be complex, but in practice, Xingyi is a pretty straightforward style (no pun intended, but there it is). One gathers energy then surges forward with a burst of speed and power, utilizing simultaneous attack and defense to overcome the enemy. It doesn't contain a lot of whirling or super-complex movements, just a total frontal total assault. I'm not saying you can learn it from these books, but you just might be able to.

Notes

1 Kennedy, Brian and Elizabeth Guo. *Chinese Martial Arts Training Manuals: A Historical Survey.* (Blue Snake Books, 2005) p. 65.
2 Kennedy & Guo. p. 87.

The Correct Path of Yiquan

By Wang Xiangzhai
(Originally published 1929. *Brennan Translations*, 2016, 25 pages)

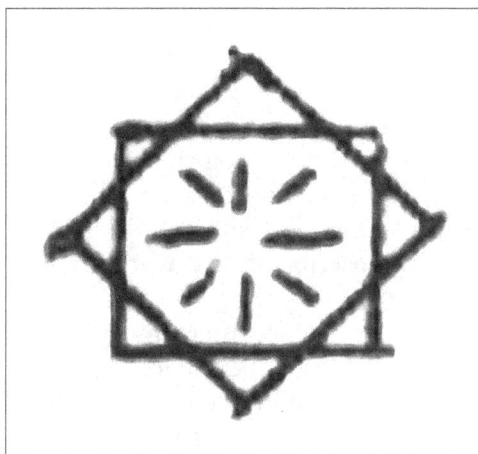

When you read a title like the one for this book, you have to wonder if the book really does aim the reader on the correct path to the art in question. With this book, though, you don't have to wonder. The author, Wang Zianghai (Wang Xiangzhai, 1885-1963), is the one who created Yiquan— or perhaps a better way to say it is that he distilled Yiquan following several decades of intensive practice, study, and research of the martial arts —not to mention practical fighting experience. And as you will see, I do mean distilled.

Wang began his martial arts career as a child under the famous Xingyi master, Guo Yunshen, who was a friend of Wang's family, proving it's nice to have family friends like that. As a young adult, Wang joined the military, then later at age thirty-three, he traveled the length and breadth of China, studying martial arts with masters of Xingyi, Southern White Crane, and Taiji, among many others. At the conclusion of his journey, he publicly declared:

> I have traveled across the country in research, engaging over a thousand people in martial combat. There have been only 2.5 people I could not defeat.

Presumably he lost to two and the .5 was a draw.

Wang moved to Beijing, where he established himself among the famous masters there and in Tianjin and Shanghai. In Beijing, he became friends with many notable masters of diverse styles, and more importantly, he began teaching his own distillation of the Chinese martial arts, which he named Yiquan. It has since also been called Dachengquan, which means "Great Achievement Boxing." He also is notable as one of the first teachers to publicly teach the chi kung called, among other names, Standing Post, Standing Tree, or Pole Standing. This was the first exercise taught to him by Master Guo, who made him hold the posture for hours.

Yiquan is sometimes termed a non-style fighting style. The name means "Intent Boxing," with the "Yi/intent" part meaning exactly the same as the "yi" or "i" in Xingyi/Xing-i. In the mid 1920, Wang came to the conclusion that Xingyi movements were too complex, turning the art more toward the external than the internal. To remedy that, he taught Xingyiquan without the Xing, or form—thus, Yiquan.

To describe his art, Wang wrote:

> In silence there must be movement, and in motion, there must be silence.
> A small movement is better than a big, no movement is better than a small, and silence is all movement's mother.
> In movement, you should be like a dragon or a tiger.
> In non-movement, you should be like a Buddha.

Originally, Yiquan had a sort of form that was soon whittled down to eight basic postures. These remain the basis of the art, but Wang continued refining his personal expression of Yiquan until he was teaching only one posture, claiming that only those who can grasp the one state and keep it are able to adequately move with it. This is much like Aikido master Koichi Tohei's "single point concentration." Wang's own teachings eventually became so abstruse that few could understand them. (Tohei, like Wang, believed his art of Aikido had become too physical, losing the internal energy that gave it power. He, too, broke away from his art's parent organization to establish his own school in an effort to reinstate the importance of internal energy to the martial arts. See Volume I of this series for a review of Tohei's *The Book of Ki.*)

This from the *Wikipedia* article on Yiquan:

> Yiquan is essentially formless, containing no fixed sets of fighting movements or techniques. Instead, focus is put on developing one's natural movement and fighting abilities through a system of training methods and concepts, working to improve the perception of one's body, its movement, and of force. Yiquan is also set apart from other Eastern martial art in that traditional concepts like qi, meridians, dantien, etc., are omitted, the reason being that understanding one's true nature happens in the present, and that preconceptions of any sort block this process.

Reading Wang's book, it's easy to see that Yiquan was developed primarily from Xingyi, yet aside from certain aspects, the book could equally be a Taiji manual since many of the precepts are similar. Indeed, watching Yiquan in action, it seems to be mostly a combination of Xingyi and a small-frame Taiji style, such as Wu Family or Northern Wu, because the applications tend to be short, highly focused, and jolting.

However, unlike either Xingyi or Taiji, Yiquan doesn't rely on forms, as noted above. Instead, the main practice is Standing Post, which is done in various configurations, with several other more complex stances (Bow Stance, for example) fleshing in things. The stance training is garnished with several light martial movements done repeatedly. Throughout, however, it is not the physical training that counts but the mental aspect of learning how to settle the body in such a way that it can be launched in any direction with full and focused force.

This makes me wonder how Yiquan folks stay in physically good shape. I did see one *Youtube* video of a Yiquan exponent teaching the well-known external chi kung known as the Eight Pieces of Brocade, but doing only that is not going to keep you physically in shape, either. Maybe Yiquan practitioners simply do other exercises to take care of what Yiquan does not. Taiji people have to do the same thing, but to a much lesser extent due to the physical exercise inherently built into Taiji forms.

The Correct Path of Yiquan begins with a preface in which the author give the historical background and philosophical reasoning behind the martial arts. An intelligent, well-read, and much traveled man, Wang also waxes eloquent on the failings of martial artists in what also could be a general indictment of negative human proclivities.

> [People] are no longer willing to use such wisdom [of knowledge gained] to seek what is truly great, and it has unfortunately become customary in recent years to incline toward what is inferior. Instead of striving for real life, they pursue empty fads. They pursue personal gain rather than self-knowledge. In imitation of corrupt literature, they seek power in order to get ahead, pages full of nonsense tricking them with illusions.

The first chapter covers, naturally, Standing Post, since this is the foundation of the art.

> In the beginning of the training, there are numerous standing methods, such as Descending Dragon Stance, Crouching Tiger Stance, Pointer Stance, Three-Realms Stance, and so on. The complexity gives way to simplicity as you take the strong points of each stance and merge them into one, called Primordial Stance. It is helpful for generating power and useful for actual fighting. It is training for mastery of both attack and defense, and for energy circulation. After just ten days of training, it will naturally produce results so marvelous that words cannot describe them.

The next chapter concerns training the sinews and bones. This section does not try to teach a method. Instead, it is primarily a catalog of Yiquan precepts along with a few pointers to improve technique. Here are just a few examples among many:

> Extending the sinews of your neck wrists, and ankles, the muscles of your whole body are thus opened up.

The six centers (the heart of the palms, the Bubbling Wells in the soles of the feet, the solar plexus, and the crown of the head) match each other.

Your joints are like the curve of a bow. Your sinews stretch like bowstrings. Wielding energy is like the tautness of the bowstrings. Send your hand out as though loosing an arrow.

Applying power is the subject of the next chapter. Wang begins with:

Effectiveness in martial arts depends on having power. Methods of applying power do not go beyond hardness and softness, squareness and roundness. Hardness is straightness. Softness is lively. Straightness is extended long, having a force of attack and defense. Softness has a shorter range, having a force that is sudden and elastic. Hard power seems to have a squareness. Soft power is externally square but internally round.

In other words, seek the straight in the curved and the curved in the straight. Wang then describes several permutations of how these aspects combine and specific ways to produce martial effect.

The author then goes into "training and cultivating the energy." Since the concept and energy of chi do not apply in Yiquan, I'm at a loss what to make of this chapter, since the energy Wang seeks to cultivate is powered by correct breathing and is concentrated in the "field of elixir," or the tantien, just as chi is powered and stored. But maybe the following will clarify matters a little. Taiji folks—and practitioners of other internal martial arts—are familiar with the concept of fa jin, or the sudden release of internal energy, either as a surging force or as a sharp and penetrating jolt or strike. Yiquan's complementary concept is fa li, or the sudden release of external strength.

In the following chapter, Wang delves into the Five Elements theory of Chinese philosophy. This is particularly germane since, just as Taiji takes its psychophysical basis from the taijitu (the tai chi symbol), Xingyi and Yiquan take it from the Five Elements theory. According to this theory, each of the five elements (water, wood, metal, fire, and earth) destroys one of the other elements and is, in turn, created by another. Water beats fire, fire beats wood, and so forth, with each of the elements being tied, in one way or another, to specific Xingyi movements or techniques. But Wang's not having it, saying that locking a fighting style into a specific set of call-and-response movements hampers that style by making it rigid and unable to respond to factors outside its usual set of stimuli. He was, after all, an early exponent of mixed martial arts and using what works, no matter what style it comes from.

But Wang's criticism of the Five Elements as applied to fighting doesn't mean that he doesn't find value in it. The way he takes it is that each of the Five Elements displays a particular strength that, working together with the others, produces the best and broadest range of martial force and agility.

> With every action, always have these five kinds of strength. This is the method of the "five elements merging into one." Whenever you are not moving, your whole body has a consistent strength, but whenever you are moving, there is everywhere, large and small joints alike, a duality of contending strength above and below, forward and back, left and right. In this way, you can gain the combined strength of your whole body.

The "Six Unions" come next, though Wang does little more than describe them in cursory terms.

> Mind is united with the intention, the intention united with the energy, and the energy united with the power. These are the three internal unions. The hand is united with the foot, the elbow united with the knee, and the shoulder united with the hip. These are there three external unions.

Taiji folks will readily see from this quote what I mean by saying this is much a Taiji manual as it is one for Yiquan.

Next comes a chapter titled, "Poetic Instructions." These instructions are basically one-liners that contain more precepts of Yiquan—very often applicable to other martial arts, as well. Further concentrate your mind, let sincerity course through your whole body, punches go out like meteors, and the head top is like a hanging chime are just a few of them. They're all worthwhile to consider.

Sparring tips is the subject of the following chapter. As stated above, Yiquan does not involve itself in specific sets of attack-and-response, so obviously, Wang does not display specific techniques. That would be futile, he says. "As there are countless transformations, they are impossible to fully describe." Instead, relaxation and going with the flow are paramount, followed by decisive strikes, throws, or joint locks.

This chapter is primarily a catalog of methods and precepts of the art. Most would be at home in a Taiji manual, but there are nuances here not normally encountered in martial arts literature, prompted, no doubt by the author's extensive practical martial experience coupled with his intelligence. I'm not going to try to list them or give examples, except for this one, which seems important:

> To win, all four limbs have to work in unison. To lose, all it takes is doubt.

Yiquan's limited repertoire of techniques are divided into two categories: Dragon and Tiger. Of the Dragon, Wang writes:

> The things it can do: stretch or shrink, can be hard or soft, can ascend and descend, can disappear and appear. In stillness it is like a mountain. When moving, it is like the wind.

Of the Tiger, he says:

> Adopt its nature and strive for its strength. Horizontally cross, vertically strike, climbing the mountain with both claws. Fiercely advance and fiercely retreat. Do lunging pounces and then short-range techniques. As though tearing prey, seem to shake your head, like a cat catching a mouse. Press up your head top and seize with your claws, rousing your whole body.

He goes on:

To sum up, the two methods of dragon and tiger are exercised without choreographed techniques. The posture is like a tiger running a thousand miles. The energy is like a dragon flying three times as far. The power finishes without the intention of finishing. And when the intention finishes, the spirit continues.

"The Correct Path of Yiquan" is the title of the final, brief chapter, which sums up the art and gives a few more pointers.

The correct path of Yiquan is nothing more than the "three classical techniques" and the two energies of dragon and tiger. While the energies of dragon and tiger are for skill building, the three techniques are for fighting. They are: stamping, drilling, and wrapping.

All three of these are types of punches that Wang describes, though not in any detail.

That's the end of the book's main text, but there is appended a short article Wang published in the Chinese periodical, *Martial Arts United Monthly*, in 1935. In it, he expounds on the need to practice martial arts, not just for the good of the body, but for the good of the body politic. But in doing so, one must approach practice correctly.

In fact, the true teaching in martial arts is simply to strive to conform to principles. The complexity or simplicity of a posture is not important. The beauty or ugliness of a movement is not important. Complex or simple, beautiful or ugly—these are not absolutes. Although a posture may appear complex, the action inside may actually be simple, and although a posture may appear simple, the action inside may actually be complex. What is within a posture is difficult to discuss because answers cannot be sought based on external appearances. What the world deems beautiful may in substance actually be ugly, and what the world deems ugly may in substance actually be beautiful.

Thanks again to translator Paul Brennan for yet another significant contribution to martial arts literature in English-language versions.

Notes

* Facts regarding Wang Zianghai and Yiquan used in this review originated in two *Wikipedia* articles:

"Wang Xiangzhai," https://en.wikipedia.org/wiki/Wang_Xiangzhai

"Yiquan," https://en.wikipedia.org/wiki/Yiquan

The Art of Xingyi Boxing

Li Jianqiu
(Originally published 1919/1922. *Brennan Translations*, 2013/2020, 34/54 pages)

The Art of Xingyi Boxing by Li Jianqiu went through two editions—1919 and 1922. Translator Paul Brennan breaks the book into two volumes. The first is of the original 1919 edition, and the second covers only the expanded versions of chapters three and four that appeared in the second edition, plus an extra foreword and some commemorative calligraphy that also appeared in the second edition. I'm going to take this as a single book, but I'll cover the original edition first and then return to the second edition's additions.

The several obligatory prefaces of the type that introduce many Chinese Republican Era martial arts manuals appear here, too, without uniqueness. The author's preface delves into Xingyi history and his own instruction in the art.

Preliminary remarks follow in which Li superficially describes the art of Xingyi. He writes:

> In former times, Guo Yunshen specialized in Xingyi, and his specialty was striking opponents with the "crashing" technique, which indicates that what makes ordinary boxing arts inferior to Xingyi Boxing is that they are flowery and are hardly useful.

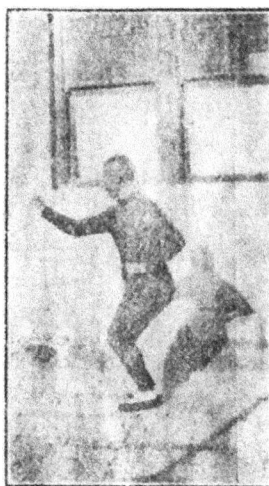

He also states:

> For those who do not engage in the two-person sets, you must when sparring not be restricted to a fixed fighting method, even though the fighting methods are written down in fixed texts. Once you are truly capable with the five elements and have something of a foundation, drill the techniques with a partner. All sorts of wonderful things can be obtained in this way, which are not necessary to record in this book.

He also says that the purpose of training in techniques is only partly to train and condition the body. The other, and perhaps more important reason is to comprehend the theory, which is more abstruse than the physical motions.

Chapter one covers the use of the boxing arts, which, the author says, is mostly to strengthen and train the body. More specifically, Xingyi, he says, is superior to other boxing arts because it is direct and easy to learn.

The next chapter is on Xingyi's fundamental Five Elements techniques. They are:

1) Chopping
2) Crashing
3) Drilling
4) Blasting
5) Crossing

Each is treated to one or more paragraphs of explanation, but as translator Brennan points out:

> [These] are not actually explanations of how to perform them, simply additional points to improve their performance.

Next, the author presents a "form," though it isn't really a form and there isn't any real instruction. Instead, it is a twelve-movement exercise in which the techniques are linked together in a continuous advance/retreat set. There is no explanatory texts and there are no photos, just a list of the techniques in order. We'll come back to these last two chapters below when we look at them in the revised edition.

Chapter five is on the deeper meaning of Xingyi. In it, Li goes into how the physical aspects of the art are bolstered and empowered by intent, and how that positively impacts health. Xingyi's four constant essentials are next.

1) Your mouth is closed, tongue touching the upper palate, saliva is generated, and is then swallowed.
2) Wrap your elbows, hang your shoulders, swell your belly, and open your chest.
3) Your legs squeeze toward each other and your toes grab the ground.
4). Your eyes should be bright and alert.

Xingyi's strong points are featured next. Here, the author compares Xingyi and "ordinary boxing arts." Those latter, he says, are merely physical movements:

> We often see practitioners of ordinary boxing arts spinning and leaping, and whenever they kick at opponents, it is nothing more than pretty. This cannot be considered anything more than a kind of exercise and is not adequate for fighting. I would be exhausting myself while the opponent takes his ease, endangering myself while the opponent rests in a position of safety. During a fight, if you feel you are already incapable of being stable, why would you then take away one of your feet to kick at opponent? If you kick but are not balanced, you are sure to lose. It is enough to quietly observed the opponent's actions and gauge how to respond. Why jump around and wear yourself out? Xingyi is without these kinds of useless actions.

In other words, Xingyi utilizes direct and targeted actions from a firm foundation. More philosophy, precepts, and methodology follow, with the author discoursing on a number of topics germane to the art—really too much to easily summarize. Besides, why take it from me when you can read the manual for yourself? Suffice it to say that Li states that the essentials of Xingyi boxing are:

1) Unification
2) Duality
3) Triple Sectioning
4) The Four Antennas
5) The five organs and their associations
6) The Six and More Unions
7) Seven advancing as one
8) Body Methods
9) Stepping principles

Each of these is given plenty of explication. The final chapter is on fighting principles. These mostly are tips to take into account when facing or engaging in confrontation rather than specific attack/response techniques.

The second edition of the book led off with a preface that is just like the other prefaces. This is followed by eleven pages of inscriptions to the author, the book, the art, concepts of the martial arts, and the health of the nation.

This is followed by the revised Chapter Three, in which the five techniques are give a far more thorough rendering, complete with explanatory text and okay photos—usually several for each technique. This is a vast improvement over the same chapter in the first edition, though you might want to take both into account for a more thorough understanding of the movements.

Ditto for the revised Chapter Four. Where the first edition simply presented a list of how the techniques are strung together into a continuous form, the second provides textual instructions and photos, giving life to the bare list's paucity.

I don't practice Xingyi, though I have played around with it a little, but this seems like a pretty good manual for the art. It fairly thoroughly presents the background information and precepts and methodology, and probably would be of interest to most Xingyi practitioners.

PART III

Bagua

Pa-kua
Chinese Boxing for Fitness and Self-Defense

by Robert W. Smith
(Kodansha International, Ltd., 1967, 160 pages)

In his introduction to *Pa-kua: Chinese Boxing for Fitness and Self-Defense,* author Robert W. Smith makes an important statement:

> Chinese books on Pa-kua boxing lay great stress on philosophical aspects which most Westerners would stamp as mysticism. My eschewing of most of these does not mean I disbelieve them. It merely means that I do not think a beginning text written for the Western reader is the place for philosophy—that too much philosophy would obfuscate material which by its very nature is difficult to present.

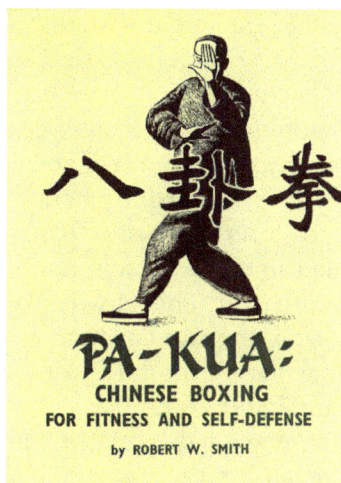

Pa-kua may be a beginner's manual, presenting basic background and instructional material, but it has historical significance, being the first book in English on the subject. Indeed, the author states that it is the first non-Chinese book on Bagua. This fact should almost be a given considering the author. Robert W. Smith was one of the earliest Westerners to widely promote the Asian martial arts in the West. His many books on the subject, under his own name and pseudonyms, would have dominated any English-language martial arts library prior to 1980. To my knowledge, his only rivals in this aspect would have been Bruce Tegnér and Donn F. Draeger. (See Volume I of this series for a review of Smith's autobiography, *Martial Musings: A Portrayal of Martial Arts in the Twentieth Century*.)

Despite Smith's demurring on the topic of philosophy, he opens the book with a historical section that includes the philosophy behind Bagua. This lies in the *I-Ching* and the resulting bagua diagram of the eight basic trigrams arranged in a circle. The history itself is amusing in that the origin of Bagua, like the origin of Taiji and Xingyi, is shrouded in time, though all three arts were reputedly created and disseminated by mysterious Taoist monks living in remote mountains. Apparently Bagua, like Taiji and Xingyi, is a gift presented to humankind directly from the Tao.

The first historical person associated with the art was Tung Haichuan (1798–1879), the student of Bagua's mysterious Taoist monk founder. Tung became famous in Beijing, and there was challenged by Kuo Yunshen, a Xingyi exponent who had killed men with his "crushing hand." The duel lasted two days and ended in a crushing defeat for Kuo. Kuo was so impressed that he and Tung became fast friends, and they agreed that their students should learn both arts. This is why Bagua and Xingyi often are coupled, and indeed, the circular nature of the former is complemented by the linear nature of the latter, and vice versa. Smith then takes us through time and a number of other masters who took up and further disseminated the art. Included are some amusing stories—legends—regarding the fantastic abilities of Tung and his successors.

Chapter two introduces what Smith calls a "beginning method." This is not the characteristic walking of the circle usually associated with Bagua but a more simplified series of eighteen independent exercises whose postures embody given martial movement patterns. In these, the feet tend to remain firmly rooted, and there is little stepping. These movements, Smith admits, are not classical Bagua and are more linear in nature, showing the influence of Xingyi. Most of the movements are presented in series of four to eight photos, and some are accompanied by secondary photos showing Smith applying the movements on an opponent. Striking dominates these movements, but there are a few sweeps and throws. The photos are clear and of adequate size.

The movements are not linked in the descriptions, but Smith later states that the practitioner should master the movements on both sides and then strive to link them into a flowing sequence, performing four in one direction, then four in the opposite direction, and so on.

The next chapter presents the classical Bagua circling method and modifications. One of the chief differences between the exercises described previously and the circling method is the application of strength. The Xingyi-like movements emphasize vertical strength while the circling method emphasizes horizontal strength. Before going into the instruction on the circling method, Smith presents twenty pages relating the principles of the art as related to him by his teacher, Kuo Fengchih.

This advice includes the concepts of relaxation and slowness, using the mind, breathing, the use of strength, and the link between substance and function, among others. Each point is expanded on, winding up with the concept of circle-walking as a training tool.

The instructions for the circle-walking begin with the single-palm change before moving on to the double-palm change, snake posture, lion posture, standing palm, and dragon posture. Each style is defined in clear text that is accompanied by good photos and foot-stepping patterns.

I've only practiced Bagua a little, and I don't have many books on the subject, so I don't have a strong enough knowledge of the art to objectively assess the quality of the material. But Smith was an experienced, energetic, and perceptive student of the Chinese martial arts, and his postures look pretty good to me. Plus, the information he presents in his various books usually is solidly based, and this one seems to be no different. So, all-in-all, this seminal English-language text on Bagua is pretty good at conveying the basics of the history, principles, and techniques of the art. Recommended.

Bagua Palming and Qinna Photos

By Chen Weiming
(Originally published by the Achieving Softness Boxing Society, 1937. *Brennan Translations*, 2020, 64 pages)

Chen Weiming was reputedly Yang Chengfu's most accomplished student, but he also learned Bagua and Xingyi from Sun Lutang. *Bagua Palming* is only one of his several books on the internal martial arts, many of them reviewed in this series.

The book leads off with three short introductions, one by Chen and two by students. Chen's provides a touch of his martial arts background, a few sentences on Bagua's history, and a couple of more on the genesis of this book. The two by his students contain mostly praise for Chen.

Then it's on to the instruction section, which consists entirely of photos without instructional text. Chen states that his intention is to provide illustrations for Sun Lutang's *A Study of Bagua Boxing*, although that book has a nearly full set of photos accompanied by instructional text. Chen's photos are larger and better-reproduced, but they might be slightly confusing at first glance for a couple of reasons.

First, the names of the movements are completely different. Where Sun uses poetic names throughout, such as "Blue Dragon Turns Its Body," Chen uses the more common terminology: "Single Palm Change." The second potential confusion is that many of Chen's photos show the movements from the opposite side com-

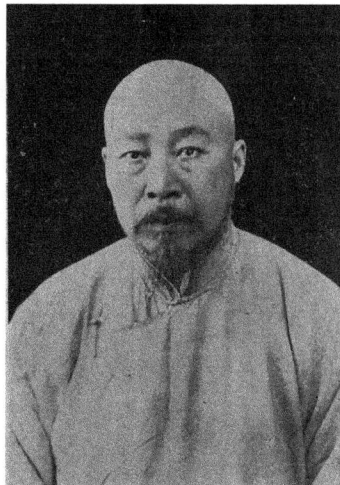

pared to photos of Sun in the same postures. But I'm thinking that might not be a bad thing since the sequence is the same, and using the two books together would allow the reader to see most of the movements from different perspectives.

Following the form instruction section, Chen demonstrates some of the movements' applications in the form of Qinna (Chin-na). As with the form instruction photos, the Qinna photos have no accompanying written instructions; however, the shots are clear enough to see what Chen is doing to his opponent. The book winds up with two short biographical sketches on Sun Lutang

Chen Weiming was an important contributor to the internal martial arts, and he left a number of books in which he attempted to explain aspects of the internal martial arts to a wide audience. He largely succeeded, even with this text-light book, in which the photos are the really valuable resource.

A Concise Book of Bagua Palming

By Yin Yuzhang
(Originally published in 1932. *Brennan Translations*, 2017, 54 pages)

Yin Yuzhang was the fourth son of Yin Fu, a prominent Yin Style Bagua practitioner, and a noted master in his own right. Yin Style is noted for having eight animal forms, and it also employs several unorthodox methodologies, including Penetrating Palm and Backhand systems. The Bagua animals forms, alone, contain, the author says, 448 unique strikes, and to those may be added a number of others from the Penetrating Palm and Backhand systems.[1]

A foreword by Yin Xuehuang extols the virtues of the Chinese martial arts and the author, and a preface by Hu Ruoyu does much the same, as does the second preface by Wan Yongshou. The third preface, by Wang Qintang goes a little farther, philosophizing on the development of the martial arts, the character they can impart, and the growing public enthusiasm for them.

Next comes introductory remarks by the author. In short snippets, he discusses the purpose of the book, the basics of Bagua and circle-walking, and a few other precepts. A few paragraphs follow on the history of the art, including its origins in an anonymous old monk living in the mountains who taught his circling art to Dong Haichuan. Dong then began teaching others, and now, the Bagua umbrella covers several branches of the art.

In a longer introduction to Bagua, Yin describes the art in greater detail, including precepts and basic methodology. Included

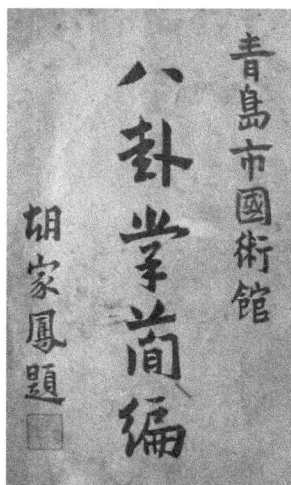

are discussions of the functioning of various body parts, alignments, walking the circle, chi, breathing, and basic tactics. None of this is deep, but it is all valid.

Then comes the form instruction section, which takes up almost all of the remainder of the book. In it are good textual instructions and photos of middling quality. It might be possible to learn some martial arts forms or katas from books, but really…. Bagua? With all its twisting and turning? Even so, Bagua enthusiasts might benefit from perusing this section.

The book closes with a short conclusion that encourages the reader to practice to achieve the full benefits of Bagua, and a short postscript by Bao Ruiyuan that says nothing more than do the several prefaces.

This is a basic Bagua manual by an acknowledged expert. While it might not have much to offer practitioners of other styles, it should be in the collection of Bagua folks.

Notes
1 "Yin Style Baguazhang." *Wikipedia*, https://en.wikipedia.org/wiki/Yin_Style_Baguazhang

PART IV

Liuhebafa
Zimen Boxing
Four-Section Boxing

A Study of Liuhebafa Boxing

By Chen Yiren
(Original publication Hong Kong, 1969, *Brennan Translations*, 2021,
  196 pages)

Liuhebafa Boxing is a lesser-known internal style whose name literally means "Six Harmonies Eight Methods Boxing." It also is known colloquially as "Water Boxing" for its characteristic flowing form that somewhat resembles Taiji. The author also refers to it as the Hibernating Dragon Art, and it has characteristics of the other internal arts of Bagua, Xingyi, and Yiquan.[1] In fact, until scholarship helped clear up the matter, it was thought to be derived from Taiji, though that notion has since been invalidated through historical research. Apparently it is a case of parallel development, thought there might have been some cross-fertilization. The system consists of bare-hand and weapons forms and several methods of chi kung.

六合八法

張之江書於滬濱

As with all of the Chinese internal martial arts, the roots of Liuhebafa are lost to time; however, its historical creation is credited to Chen Tuan (allegedly 871–989).[2] (Chen Yiren sometimes refers to Chen Tuan as Chen Xiyi.) Chen also supposedly is associated with the Taiji Ruler, also called Taiji Bang, a one-foot stick used to aid in energy manipulation. (See a review of *Tai Chi Bang*, by Jesse Tsao, later in this volume.)

Like almost all creators of internal martial styles, Chen was a Taoist monk who resided for a time in the Wudang Mountains. He was well-educated and learned, and in addition to being conversant

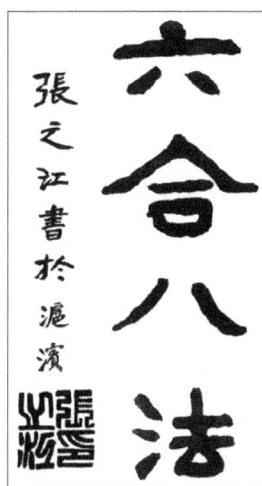

with the Classics, history, medicine, astronomy, and geography, he also was a poet. As a thinker, he had a profound influence both real and mythic on later generations.

A Study of Liuhebafa Boxing is a more-than-adequate summation of the art by a skilled expert, and the book opens with a dozen poems and a handful of prefaces by others to that effect. The last preface, by the author, relates how he became involved in the martial arts and lays out his lineage. This includes his teachers, his pupils, his writings, and his mastery of the martial arts—particularly Liuhebafa, which he learned from Wu Yihui. Brief remarks then characterize the art, saying that is has never before been shared publicly, and that it emphasizes virtue rather than force.

> The movements must be slow, gentle, smooth, comfortable, and be a single flow from beginning to end. The elbows should constantly be slightly bent and hanging down. There has to be vertical alignment between the shoulders and hips, elbows and knees, hands and feet. There must be both hardness and softness, emptiness and fullness. Stay alert and adaptable. Every movement should be filled with significance.

A chapter on the origins of Liuhebafa comes next. It is in three parts, the first and third by Chen's teacher, Wu Yihui, and the middle one is by the author. I'm not sure why Chen had Wu write some of this. Perhaps Chen was honoring Wu by giving him a place in the book. Or maybe Wu knew the historical material better than Chen. A more likely scenario is that the section that Chen writes is about Wu, relieving Wu of the task of self-promotion. In any case, the history begins with the art's creator, Chen Tuan, and runs from his childhood to his death. It is something like the usual story of a son expected to rise in academic studies but who, instead, gravitates toward the martial arts and spiritual pursuits.

The account moves on to Chen's teacher, Wu Yihui, who is credited with opening the teaching of Liuhebafa to the general public. Wu's life is given solid treatment, and he cuts an impressive figure as martial artist, military leader, and scholar. The third historical section gives a summation of the art.

The next chapter is titled, "Boxing Secrets in Five-Character Lines." As this implies, these are short but pithy statements, sometimes couched poetically, on the precepts and methodology of Liuhebafa. These would be at home in just about any book on any internal style, and some of them are rather witty:

> Look upon your ability as though you do indeed have ability. However, if you are still inexperienced in the art, do not try your luck against opponents.

These statements occupy nine pages, then it's on to more inscriptions by other writers before Chen gets down to brass tacks by listing a number of important points to keep in mind regarding Liuhebafa.

> The essence of our Mind and Intention art is that the six unions provide the theory and the eight methods provide the function.

The Six Unions are:

1) Body unites with mind.
2) Mind unites with intention.
3) Intention unites with energy.
4) Energy unites with spirit.
5) Spirit unites with movement.
6) Movement unites with void.

Some readers will notice a definite difference between this list and the Six Unions that are normally listed in internal martial arts manuals:

External unions
   1) Hand united with foot.
   2) Elbow united with knee.
   3) Shoulder united with hip.
Internal unions
   4) Mind united with intent.
   5) Intent united with energy.
   6) Energy united with power.

Chen's Eight Methods are:

1) Energy: Use concentration of spirit to direct the flow of energy.
2) Bone: Use your skeletal structure to store power.
3) Shape: Constantly transform, mimicking nature and other people.
4) Follow: Accommodate and go along with the opponent's movements.
5) Ascend: Suspend your head top, producing a feeling of floating in midair.
6) Return: Go back and forth, reversing everything the opponent is trying to do so that it rebounds on him.
7) Rein in: Settle into quietude and maintain emptiness.
8) Conceal: Disappear and hide what you are about to do.

These points are not elaborated on, but the next chapter, "Boxing Secrets in Five-Character Lines," provides a more thorough analysis of the aforementioned. It begins with the statement:

> In this boxing art, the most important thing is internal power, but there is also value in the methods. The highest level is to understand power and to know the methods. The middle level is to understand power but be without methods. The lowest level is to be without methods and have no understanding of power. Understanding power is difficult. Knowing the methods is also difficult. Therefore this boxing art is difficult to learn, but even more difficult to understand.

Chen then goes over the major joints of the body, body alignment, and how the energy is to be moved successively through the joints to fill the entire the body. But, the author stresses, while one should pay attention to all of this, one must not become "stuck" by adhering too closely to patterns. Flexibility of both mind and body are essential, and the ultimate state is to have the mind fundamentally empty of methods.

A discussion of the Liuhebafa solo set comes next, and this is more about general principles rather than specific movements. Chen then discusses Liuhebafa's internal theories, which pretty much coincide with similar theories about Taiji. This mostly is an overview, with subsections titled, "The Primal Source," "Memory and Understanding," "Caverns Where Energy Is Transformed," "Dragon and Tiger," "Fire and Water," "Primordial Active Energy," and "Naturalness." This material, though well-enough explained, can be somewhat abstruse.

The last, and longest, section of the book—about 150 pages—contains the form instruction. Each movement is described in words and a sequence of photos. The text is adequate, and the photos are more than adequate, showing several phases of each movement. The book closes with a short afterword by another writer that sums up the book.

This is a worthwhile introduction to Liuhebafa for those interested in learning the art or those just plain interested in the various Chinese internal martial arts. Water Boxing is a style not often seen, but that doesn't mean it shouldn't be.

Notes

1 "Liuhebafa." *Wikipedia*, https://en.wikipedia.org/wiki/Liuhebafa.
2. "Chen Tunan." *Wikipedia*, https://en.wikipedia.org/wiki/Chen_Tuan.

Authentic Zimen Boxing
Including Secret Records of Injury Medicines

By Hu Yusheng
(Originally published by the Central Martial Arts Institute, 1933.
Brennan Translations, 2014, 112 pages)

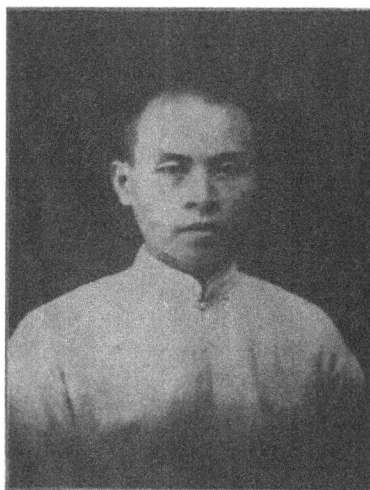

Some martial arts employ forms/ kata to teach the repertoire of that particular art. Others simply practice repetitive drills that teach the martial techniques without stringing them into forms. And at least one I've reviewed in this series uses minimal forms or techniques, but mostly only Standing Post and mental intent. Zimen seems to be a combination of technique drills that eventually can be put together into forms.

Zimen is a rather rare style that also is known as a Ruan Men (Soft Gate/Internal) martial art and is now practiced mostly in the Jiangxi Province of China's south-central plains. It was created around 300 years ago by Yu Kerang, who was native to the province. The style consists of various fast and powerful unbalancing combat methods, and it also includes Dim Mak among its skills. The style's genesis parallels that of Taiji for a time, but diverged when Taiji largely divested itself of deadly point-striking techniques, while Zimen continued with them. For more information on Zimenquan, check out the Taiping Institute page on the art.[1]

Authentic Zimen Boxing begins with a brief biography of the author's teacher, Zen Master Kexiu, by Rao Caorong. Rao characterizes him thus:

> The more refined his skill became, the more density his internal power developed. When he arrived at Yanshan, challengers came to visit him, to who he was always polite, never seeking to boost his reputation through these matches nor boasting of his victories. His body appears lame and weak, and he is not at all grand in stature, but when he sends power to his fingertips, he can make a hole in a wall. His stance is so stable, he calls for several robust men to pull his feet with ropes but stands proud and immovable. He also is proficient at trauma medicine.

A few lines from Sun Yat-sen lead into the book. Hu begins with a few comments about the book and its contents. Then comes a preface by Rao Carong, in which he performs what by now seems like a ritual bemoaning of the state of China's society and culture that is common among the prefaces of Chinese martial arts manuals of the early to mid 20th century.

This is followed by the author's preface in which he performs the usual duties of complaining about the state of the martial arts and voicing the need for a reinvigoration of the arts. He does, though, define Zimen: zi = word, men = school. This means "the school of eighteen words," so designated because of its eighteen primary techniques. He also says that very few practitioners have learned the whole art or understand it completely.

Next, Hu presents an overview of the eighteen techniques, and his descriptions make clear the loose connection to Taiji and other internal martial arts:

> A body that is extremely weak has been inadequately equipped by what is innate, and this has to be compensated for by training that is acquired. The way of filling this gap lies in cultivation expense and spirit.... Once the way of turning weakness into strength is understood, then study the eighteen techniques. What is emphasized within the techniques is the skill of tendon-based power. If the tendons are

not worked, laziness will lead to atrophy and cramping. Tendon-based power merges with health, and thus flexibility will not be held back.

The Eighteen Techniques are:

1) Testing
2) Sending
3) Aiding
4) Seizing
5) Pulling
6) Pushing
7) Crowding
8) Absorbing
9) Sticking
10) Hoisting
11) Curving
12) Inserting
13) Throwing
14) Propping
15) Rubbing
16) Scattering
17) Vanishing
18) Ejecting

Each of these is treated to a sentence or two of explanation. Next comes the "Secret of the Eight Primary Techniques," in which Ejecting, Sending, Aiding, Pulling, Pushing, Crowding, Absorbing, and Testing are further explicated as sequences of techniques. Ditto for the next two short chapters.

There is no form, so the instruction section just shows each of the eighteen techniques. Each has text instructions and a single line drawing. Following that is a chapter that is fairly unusual for martial arts manuals of the time in depicting eight ground-fighting techniques.

There follows two essays elaborating upon the subtleties of the art. The first is on maintaining willpower. In it, Hu discusses perseverance and the fact that the martial arts are as much about health as they are about fighting. He then breaks the boxing arts into two rather obvious aspects: bodily health and self-defense.

In addition to speaking about perseverance, Hu notes four things to guard against:

1) Restrain your lust.
2) Restrain your greed.
3) Abstain from alcohol.
4) Prevent illness.

The next chapter discusses preserving the essence. Essence, or internal energy, is what gives the martial artist power. Thus, Hu recommends abstaining from sex in order to prevent squandering of one's essence. From there, Hu delves into several aspects of internal energy and the kind of power that its preservation will unleash. Cultivating the internal energy is the subject of the next chapter, and Hu has this to say:

> The energy of the human body is the easiest thing to waste or spoil.

There follows a number of examples of preserving essence and wasting it. This consists of statements about essence and examples illustrated by anecdotes. Righteousness is the key to excellence in the martial arts, Hu says.

> Behaving in this way, energy will fill your body, and the Way and righteousness will soon express as noble energy. Mengzi said: "The mind leads the energy. The energy leads the body." Therefore, without the mind leading, the energy will be in chaos. With your energy in chaos, your spirit will be distracted. With your spirit distracted, your emotions will be in a panic. With your emotions panicking, hour hands will become stagnant.... Thus the cultivation of energy is greatly involved in defense against opponents, and practitioners have to understand this.

Chapter four is "Gathering Spirit." In it, Hu discusses how ample spirit can enable a person to accomplish what might seem like miracles to others. But doing such things is really just a matter of gathering and focusing the spirit on a particular task and allowing it to make the necessary movements. There is a lot in this chapter, so I'll let a few quotes suffice to exhibit the range:

> Whenever we practice these skills, we must strive to be elegant rather than imitating the imposing stature of the "valiant martial man."

> Do not have any expectation or use any effort. By not requiring it, power will come. Do not be distracted from simply feeling it. Power will manifest without any help.

> When walking, step slowly rather than quickly, with shoulders dropped rather than raised, eyes not watching more than ten feet away, hands not swaying off more than half a foot, forefingers extended rather than curled up.

There are more, on standing, sitting, lying down. The next chapter discusses taking the right path, or, making sure that your efforts are aimed at the real and genuine, not at self-satisfying mirages. Much of the concentration in this chapter focuses on remaining flexible and soft until it's necessary to be hard. Hu also discusses leverage and how the direction of power can be altered to do useful work or tasks. But he also cautions to make one's practice gradual and rational to prevent potentially serious injury.

The next chapter covers the eighteen techniques. Here, they are fully explicated and linked to the style's other movements—not so much in a form, but as a method of call-and-response. Each is defined and given a sort of ersatz application. This is involved stuff that is valuable for any martial artist, but it might resonate more for the internal stylist.

Improving one's stance is the subject of the next chapter. The author writes:

> For one whose skill is deep, his power will penetrate the ground deeply.

Next, he discusses strategy in relation to the eighteen techniques, including the rigorous stance training forced on him by his teacher. This leads into the next chapter on dispelling an opponent's force, which includes strategy as well as techniques, and several scenarios are recounted. Hu cautions against misjudging an opponent, whether he is young and seemingly wet behind the ears or old and seemingly decrepit, for neither might be what they seem. He also says:

> When applying techniques, you should focus your mind. Focusing your mind makes your brain alert. With your brain alert, you will sense things quickly. Sensing quickly, your body and hands become like springs.

"Developing Power" is the next chapter. He begins with:

> Force is like iron. Power is like steel. But if force is not trained, you will be incapable of achieving power.

From there, he discusses how force and power operate within the body. Force is physical, power is esoteric. Using force will prevent one from being able to utilize power. He gives several exercises to improve one's sense of power and to increase its strength. Sometimes, these seem a little like those horrendous training exercises you see Gordon Liu go through in his movies about the Shaolin Temple.

The following chapter is "Lightening the Body." Hu writes:

> The light-body skill has always been secret and untransmitted.

This skill refers to being able to jump high and land without a thud, to easily climb unclimbable objects such as a flagpole, and even seem to fly. He approaches these feats as credible, saying he's personally witnessed some of them, and then he describes several exercises designed to help one achieve this skill. It's more Gordon Liu training.

Hu goes into practical applications next, and he says that this is the most difficult part. The novice, he says, will fail repeatedly at first until he gains an understanding of how the dynamics of confrontation play out. As far as applications go, Hu has this to say:

> For our techniques there are no choreographed practice sets, not fixed patterns of footwork. We attack boldly when facing opponents, advancing as we please…. The movements

of our hands not restricted by prescribed ways of how techniques should follow or precede each other.

Chapter twelve is on meditation. Hu writes:

> What is valued in the martial arts is movement, but what is displayed is meditation. Why is this? Because while practicing a techniques, even if your body is externally hard, internally it would actually be brittle. You must rely on meditation to solidify internally.

He illustrates the importance of internal solidity this way:

> A glass stored away in an iron safe can withstand an attack from a stick, but give the safe a strong shake and the glass will break. Therefore we can say that unless there is solidity internally, you can perform the fierce striking of a strong person yet be unable to handle a finger strike from an expert.

The next few paragraphs describe stillness and how it enables one to sense internal energy and learn to move it inside your body for the purposes of health and emotional and spiritual well-being. As with Hu's other descriptions of important points to ponder, he illustrates these with anecdotes.

This is the end of the main text. What remains is *Secret Records of Injury Medicines*, compiled by the author. There are approximately twenty-five pages of these medical recipes, some of which are salves or unguents, while others are to be taken internally. Hu supplies the names of the medicines and the part of the body to which they are to be applied, but for the unguents, he doesn't give the actual recipes, just the ingredients. Under the rubric, "Generalized Effects of Medicines," he does give the actual recipes, but the reader should be wary since not all traditional Chinese medical cures are effective. For example, under the heading, "For livening the energy," the cure calls for consuming either monkey or tiger bones. Another recommends licorice root for strengthening tendons, although modern research has found that licorice is not good for the human male heart, and overconsumption can lead to a heart attack. To rid oneself of decrepitude, Hu recommends musk. Consumed? Applied externally? Snorted? Who can say? I think I'll stick to exercise and modern medicine, at least for the most part.

I might be able to make fun of this last chapter, but I can't about any of the rest of this interesting and valuable book. It's not going to teach you how to perform Zimen Boxing, but it'll teach you a lot about other martial matters.

Notes

1 "Zimenquan." Taiping Institute, http://taipinginstitute.com/zimenquan

Four-Section Boxing Explained

By Xu Shijin
(Originally published by Hankou Martial Arts Institute, 1935. *Brennan Translations*, 2018, 56 pages)

Xu Shijin's *Four-Section Boxing Explained* begins with an introduction titled, "Encouragement to Promote Chinese Martial Arts," by Chiang Kai-shek, which appeared as a preface to *Central Martial Arts Institute Collection of Articles* (1928). This was shortly before Chiang became actual leader of the Chinese Nationalist government. But despite the authorship, it has little more substance than most forewords in Republican Era martial arts manuals.

A preface by one of Xu's students, Liu Fu, follows, and it is pretty much another standard preface, although he does say that the form depicted in this book is a combination of Taiji, Bagua, and Xingyi. Frankly, there doesn't seem to be much Taiji in it, and it seems to be mostly Xingyi, but then I only have the photos to go by.

A second preface, this one by Liu Wenzhu, adds that author Xu was director of the Hankou Martial Arts Institute, and a third preface, by Tian Guoan, adds nothing.

Then Xu begins his text with the origins of the art and how to practice it. The art was created, he says, by Yue Fei, the famous general who supposedly created Xingyi, which explains why Four-Section Boxing most resembles that art.

Next, he discusses three things to pay attention to:

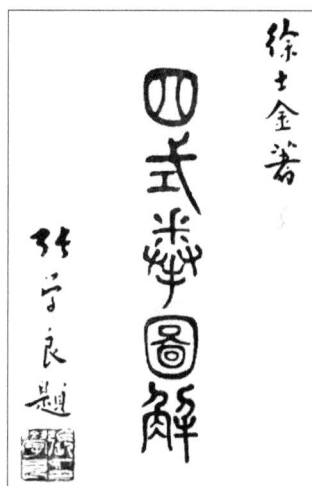

1) Before practice—Don't be hungry or full, don't think too much, and don't be angry
2) During practice—No laughing, spitting, farting
3) After practice—Do not eat or drink, do not excrete, do not lay down and sleep

The three stages of practice are next:

1) Stage 1—The movements should be soft and slow.
2) Stage 2—The movements should be more fierce and quick.
3) Stage 3—There should be hardness and softness complementing each other.

Three things to avoid in training are:

1) Do no be too certain.
2) Do no become complacent.
3) Do not give up on yourself.

After this comes the form instruction section demonstrating a thirty-seven-posture form broken into four parts It is a very upright form with no low movements or kicks. The textual instructions are adequate but do not show applications. The photos are of two types. Most are of the author, and these are pretty good though severely faded. The other photos, interspersed among those of the author, are older and are, presumably, of his teacher, who is unnamed. These older photos are almost completely useless.

The book closes with an afterword by the author that actually was written for the Central Martial Arts Institute's second National Tournament, but it contains little more than most of the prefaces.

PART V

Taiji Push Hands
Applications

Practical Use of Tai Chi Chuan
Its Application and Variation

by Yeung (Yang) Sau Chung
(Tai Chi Co., 1977, 42 pages)

Taiji folks, over the many, many years of the art, have produced some curious books, and *Practical Use of Tai Chi Chuan: Its Application and Variation* is one of them. Its length is so brief that there isn't enough room on the spine for the book's title and author.

Yeung is the son of Yang Chenfu, using an alternate spelling of the family name (Yang Zhenming and Yang Shaozhong being other names he went by). He opens this small book with a three-page exposition of Taiji that has a bit of substance, but it's relatively slight compared to what is delivered by most beginner manuals. If you want to read about Taiji's history, principles, and basic practices, you can find much, much more complete information elsewhere.

Next comes a fold-out page that contains, on one side, a series of photos of the Yang Style long form, and on the other side, a written list of the names of the movements. On the plus side, the photos are all of Yang Chengfu. You often see some of these historic photos in other books, but it's rare to see the entire sequence at one time. On the minus side, the photos are the size of postage stamps and are pretty grainy, so frankly, they're not particularly helpful. And amusingly for a book in English, the photos display right-

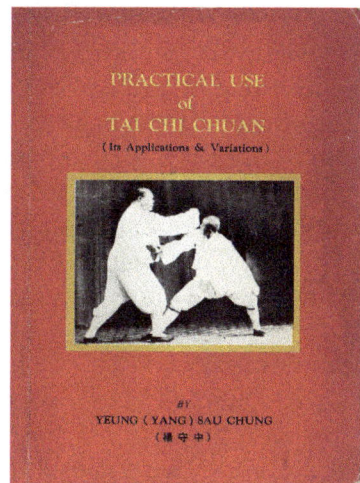

to-left, so if you're going to examine the sequence, you'll have to reverse your normal reading direction. Nor is the list on the reverse side helpful—at least for those of us who do not read or speak Chinese—as the names of the movements are all in that language, both in Romanized characters and in ideograms. This despite the fact that the movements are given English names in the pages that follow.

The rest of the book is taken up with photos and descriptions of applications from the form. The top half of each page describes an application illustrated by a photo, usually of Yang Chengfu pushing around another guy who looks a little like Chen Weiming, but I can't swear to that identification. The bottom half shows a potential follow-up action that emerges from the application pictured at the top. The photos that illustrate these are usually of Yeung Sau Chung applying the movements to several other people. All the photos of Yang Chengfu are of relatively mediocre quality, though the ones at the bottom of the page are better.

I'm not a big fan of such books. Sure, with a partner and diligence, you might be able to suss out how an applications really works, but single static photos of applications are pretty limited in describing dynamic movement. Of course, when this book first came out, we didn't have the proliferation of application videos that we now do, so maybe it was a more valuable work at the time. But not now.

If *Practical Use of Tai Chi Chuan* has any value now, it's in its presentation (poor as it is) of the sequence featuring Yang Chengfu and in the somewhat better photos of him applying Taiji to his sparring partner. My copy of this book is old, but apparently there is a newer edition with a different cover on the market. Buy it if you want or need to look at mediocre photos of Yang Chengfu's form, but don't if that isn't something that interests you.

T'ai Chi for Two
The Practice of Push Hands

by Paul Crompton
(Shambhala, 1989, 122 pages)

You might be able to learn push hands from Paul Crompton's *T'ai Chi for Two*. Maybe, though these days, you probably can learn this stuff as well or better from *Youtube* videos if you don't have someone to teach you. But instruction isn't the real value of the book despite the basically adequate descriptions of specific push hands patterns and techniques.

Instead, the best thing about this book is that it's an extended meditation that delves into the personal, interpersonal, and larger spiritual aspects of push hands. Crompton lays these out in a calm, measured tone tempered by experience. In general, he takes a no-nonsense approach that insists on the ideas that detached observation trumps desire and that letting go is the swiftest way forward.

Along the way, he delves into the implications of the taijitu (the tai chi symbol), the concept of chi, and the importance of having an empty mind, all with a healthy debunking of some of the more extravagant mythology surrounding Taiji. And the whole is peppered with stories and anecdotes to illustrate his points, making this more fun to read than his otherwise composed prose might indicate.

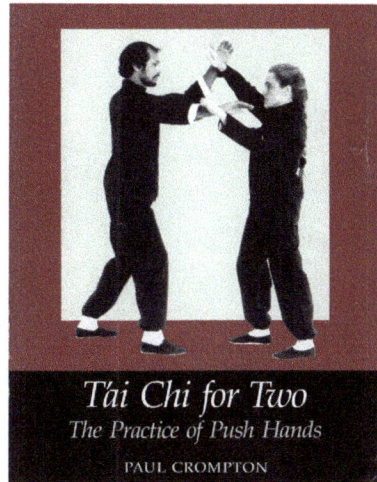

Most of the middle of the book is taken up by instructional photos and text, but even if you're not specifically interested in studying the techniques, you shouldn't skip this section but continue reading since there's a lot of interesting information tucked into it. The final chapters discuss Taoist teachings in modern terms.

This book falls somewhere between philosophy and nuts-'n-bolts, and it contains a lot of philosophical musings mixed with somewhat detailed instructional material, though it is geared more toward the beginner and intermediate student than toward the advanced one.

Wu Style Taichichuan Tuishou

by Ma Yueh-liang and Zee Wen, MD
(Shanghai Book Co., Ltd., 1986, 86 pages)

The International Wu Style Taiji Chuan Federation is one good place to find information on Wu Family Taiji, but until recently, Wu Style practitioners have had far fewer resources for information about the genesis, development, and unique characteristics of their style than Yang stylists have enjoyed. Any further elucidation, however slight, is welcome, and Ma Yuehliang's several books provide valuable information from a master close to Wu Style's origins.

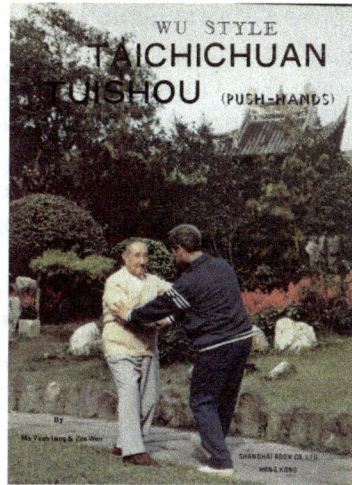

Ma Yueh-liang might not have been a blood member of the Wu family, but he not only married into it and so excelled at the art that he became famous in his own right for the skills he honed. He also is notable for being the teacher of Sophia Delza, whom he taught in the years shortly after WWII. Delza was the first person to demonstrate Taiji to the American public, to openly teach the art in the United States, and to publish a book in English on Taiji: *T'ai-Chi Ch'uan: Body and Mind in Harmony*. (Reviewed in Volume VI of this series.)

Ma was well-known for his tuishou (push hands), a skill that he apparently did not fully develop until later in life, and he directed the Shanghai Chien Chuan Tai Chi Chuan Association. He left fewer than a handful of books, but a large legacy.

The book opens with a preface by Delza, and there is a certain irony in this, though I know why it was done. Delza was one of the most prominent Taiji figures in the U.S. for many years, and practically the sole promoter of Wu Style in a Taiji sphere dominated by Yang Style. This makes her the obvious choice to write the preface. But Delza was known for promoting the exercise, artistic, and self-development aspects of Taiji rather than its martial side, so the irony rests in her prefacing a book on tuishou.

Delza's preface is followed by a forward and introduction by co-author Zee Wen. In them, he relates a pinch of history and a dash of philosophy and touches on a few of Taiji's more obvious principles. A short chapter, also by Zee, discusses in broad strokes tuishou and its relationship to practice of the Taiji form. Next is a chapter on Wu Chian-chuan (Wu Chienchuan) and the Chian-chuan Taichichuan Association, which was the name of the Wu family organization prior to World War II, during which time the Japanese occupiers of China suppressed the martial arts. The text includes biographical information on Wu Chianchuan and an outline of the formation and development of the association. The text glosses over the years of WWII but picks up after the war and states that several decades passed before the association fully rebounded. Today, Wu Family Style's many branches are subsumed under the International Wu Style Taiji Chuan Federation.

Then it's on to the body text of the book, which comprises three parts, the third being an appendix. Part one consists of five chapters, each on some aspect of Taiji or tuishou. Chapter one—"Longevity and Eternal Spring"—lays out the philosophical background of Taiji as an intimate melding of health and martial practices that trains the practitioner to utilize skill rather than brute strength. Dedicated practice produces a relaxation and stillness reaction rather than an alarm reaction, preserves physiological and mental health, and strengthens the bones. Each of these aspects are discussed over several paragraphs.

Chapter two introduces what the author calls the "Thirteen Kinetic Movements" of Taiji. These are more commonly referred to as the "Thirteen Postures" or "Thirteen Dynamics," and they form the foundation of all Taiji movements. An overview divides the Thirteen Postures into the eight directions, or Eight Gates, and the Five Steps, which are further linked to the theory of the five Chinese elements. Then the authors provide a more in-depth analysis of each of the Eight Gates and Five Steps. The descriptions are clearly stated and are generally superior to similar definitions found in other Taiji texts.

Throughout, the authors stress that the force of the practitioner's application of any of the Thirteen Postures against an opponent is completely dependent on the force applied by the opponent. In other words, the practitioner meets light force with light response and heavy force with heavier response, which makes sense in an art that utilizes the energy of the opponent to impel one's own movement.

Chapter three is titled "The Characteristics and Mechanical Fundamentals of Tuishou." It opens with a recitation of Ma's five-character motto for learning Taiji: calmness, lightness, slowness, exactness, and perseverance. Taiji is the art of using the mind rather than force, and the authors state that this does not mean that no exertion is need in combat, but that mind-concentrated force is much more powerful than physical force alone. Each of the five elements is then elucidated with similar depth that the authors gave to their discussion of the Thirteen Postures.

The next chapter defines five characteristics of Taiji: overcome hardness with softness, meet offense with calmness, win with lesser strength but superior skill, retreat in order to advance, and use circular movements. Following that, they discuss four points that illustrate the mechanical fundamentals of tuishou:

1) The rule of the center of gravity
2) The role of "coupling," which is the use of two forces moving in opposite directions to create circular movement (such as two fingers gripping a key and pushing in opposite directions to turn it in a lock)
3 & 4) Impulse and momentum, the prolongation of which produces greater internal force

Chapter four delves into the way that practiced skill accrues over time to produce what Ma calls "strength perception," but which Taiji exponents more commonly know as "sensing jing"—the ability to sense the direction, pressure, and quality of an attacking force even as it is being initiated, allowing the practitioner to deal with it in the most effective way possible. This skill, the authors state, is the root of tuishou excellence and is the result of self-cultivation rather than rote muscle memory.

Chapter five is devoted to a question-and-answer session in which Ma (and occasionally Sophia Delza) answer questions on a variety of Taiji topics, ranging from the need for correct posture to health to the characteristics of fast Taiji forms.

Part two moves away from the philosophical and into the practical, and it contains a great many photos to illustrate the points in the text. It begins with basic stances and various hand postures, then goes into specific instructions for several tuishou forms, starting with single-hand push hands with fixed steps. Double-hand with fixed steps is next, followed by thirteen variations on double-hand, fixed-step operations. Tuishou with moving steps is illustrated next, and there are six variations shown, including da lu, sometimes called the "big pulldown," though the form shown here is somewhat different than the da lu I learned. This ends the major text, leaving the book to close with an appendix containing translations of five of the Taiji Classics.

I'm not generally a fan of form-instruction material in Taiji books. Taiji and its ancillary forms such as tuishou are difficult enough to learn from a live teacher and are, I believe, practically impossible to learn from a book, even given willing participants. So, while the instructional section on tuishou is highly detailed and well illustrated, it can be easily skimmed over by the novice, who might gain little from it. But this section could be of value to folks who already are versed in tuishou and who are looking to expand their repertoire and understanding. Part one of the book, however, contains a great deal of important information that can apply to any Taiji style, not just Wu Family Taiji.

In addition, the text relates several anecdotes that highlight Ma's extraordinary skills in repelling force with movements that seem almost invisible. This section alone is worth the price of admission—if one can now afford it. I bought this book for $5 in 1986, but Amazon's website shows new copies being sold for as much as $53, though copies can also be had for under $20. The former seem to be offerings by resellers, who always jack up the price to make their profit.

Tui Shou & San Shou in T'ai Chi Ch'uan

by Yiu Kwong
(Yiu Kwong Herbalist, 1981, 160 pages)

It's tough to learn the movements of Taiji, in any of its aspects—form or push hands—from a book. Maybe not impossible, but tough. When this book on push hands came out in 1981, there were few Taiji resources aside from a couple of score of books and a handful of video tapes, which is why I bought it in the first place.

The text is presented in both Chinese and English, and the English version is very awkward. The author acknowledges this in his introduction, writing:

> This book has been 'roughly' written by me. I wish readers would excuse my misinterpretations appeared in the book which have been brought about by my low level of academy. [Sic for that whole sentence.]

The awkward writing might be excused if the information imparted is of relatively high quality, but unfortunately, that isn't the case here. The brief expository material is limited to thumbnail descriptions of the Eight Gates (Wardoff, Rollback, Press, Push, Pull/Pluck, Split, Elbow Strike, and Shoulder Strike), which the author calls "force feats." You can work through the unwieldy prose to glean what the author is saying, but you still won't get a whole lot out of the descriptions.

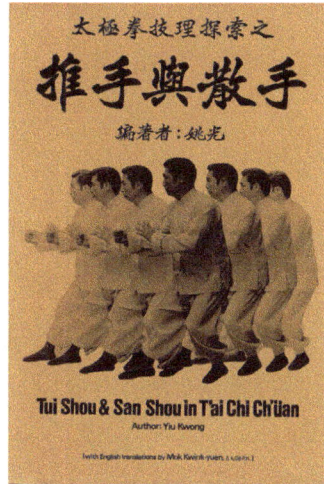

This meager introduction is out of the way by the end of page fifteen, and the remainder of the book is devoted to instructional material on several types of push hands patterns and a great many applications based on form postures. This material is not bad, per se, and might serve if you and your partner don't have a live teacher or access to videos, but just barely.

Over all, this is a pretty weak book in more than one aspect: My copy has fallen apart at the spine, and that certainly isn't from overuse. Yiu's first book, *The Research into Techniques and Reasoning of T'ai Chi Ch'uan*, is a better beginner book, though still far from the best. (Reviewed in Volume VI of this series.)

On Applying the Art

Shi Diaomei
(Originally published by the Huaxin Publishing Co., 1959. *Brennan Translations* 2021, 54 pages)

The art in question is Taiji, and this book is a thorough primer on push hands and the two push hands patterns of tui shou and san shou.

Author Shi Diaomei covers basic principles in the first chapter, discussing the need to let go of one's ego in order to respond naturally and properly. Thus, he maintains, pushing hands isn't really antagonism but cooperation. Even if the antagonist isn't trying to cooperate, the defending Taijiquanist should have enough cooperation for the both of them.

Shi touches on other aspects of push hands, such as the ideas of fixed and moving step push hands, stance (which he calls the "three-line stance), breathing, and the positions of the arms before moving on to chapters devoted to specific essentials. These are listening, neutralizing, seizing, and issuing. Each of these concepts is treated to an excellent explanation.

Then Shi goes into a chapter that breaks down a fixed-step tui shou pattern in words and photos. Push hands instructions in Taiji manuals is usually kind of pointless since it would be practically im-

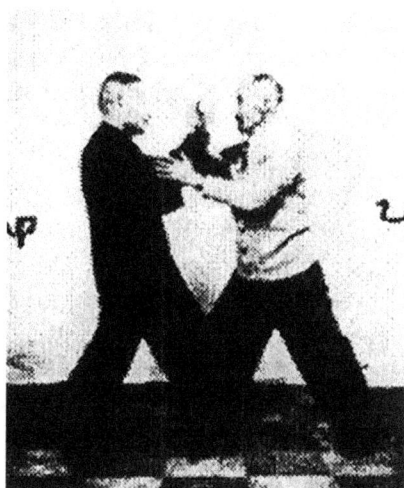

possible for most people to learn to do it from a book. Even the author acknowledges that fact:

> Pushing hands is not actually something that can be learned from a book. This is because listening, neutralizing, seizing, and issuing are too ephemeral, constantly changing from one thing to another, and so cannot be demonstrated adequately through photographs.

The text in this instruction section section is scanty, and the photos are mostly of such terrible quality that you can't tell what the two guys are actually doing. This practically useless chapter yields to a short chapter that is replete with excellent material in the form of precepts and methodologies to take into account when pushing hands.

The next chapter contains another form instruction, this one for da lu, or the "Big Rollback," which is a more vigorous push hands pattern than tui shou. After a lengthy and informative introduction to the ideas behind da lu, the author breaks down the pattern in words and photos, much as he did with tui shou, and with the same deficiencies. As with the tui shou chapter, the da lu instruction section is followed by a chapter of principles and methodologies, and as before, this material is far stronger than that in the instruction section.

The next chapter is on sparring, and it begins by giving credibility to the idea that Wang Tsung-yueh taught Taiji to the Chen family. However, Shi isn't really interested in origins, but in functionality.

> Whatever version of the [Tai Chi] boxing set you practice, regardless of whether it is derived from the old frame or new frame Chen Style, if you can apply the training and the principles, then your techniques will all have practical functions.

The author further characterizes Taiji, summing up with this:

> Within ordinary boxing manuals, there are often photos of applications. You can certainly practice according to such demonstrations. However, you should not treat these presentations of applications as being definitive, you need to experiment with applications for yourself. Without choreographed patterns, it is difficult to learn the basics. But with-

out moving on from choreographed patterns, it is difficult to progress to a high level.

The next chapter discusses applying the energies of Taiji. Shi begins by contrasting hard/external strength with soft/internal power. Then he lists the energies that can be manipulated:

1) Sticking
2) Adhering
3) Borrowing
4) Neutralizing
5) Yielding
6) Drawing In
7) Lifting
8) Seizing
9) Catching
10) Penetrating
11) Interrupting
12) Sinking
13) Opening
14) Closing
15) Wrapping
16) Shaking
17) Traversing Emptiness

Each is defined to a greater or lesser degree, but all the explanations are cogent. There is lots of good material here.

The next chapter contains forty-two verbatim statements made to the author by his teacher, Tian Zhaolin. They contain words of wisdom for those engaging in push hands, running the gamut from what to do in particular situations to concepts of neutralization to dealing with an opponent's force and more. All this is valuable stuff.

Next is a similar chapter that excerpts writing from former masters, and as with the previous section, this one is chock full of excellent material. It is, essentially, the main explanation of Taiji from Yang Chengfu's own book. Following that are two Taiji Classics written by Li Yiyu, and that is followed by a number of excerpts from Sun Lutang. (All of this latter material is excerpted from full-length works that have been reviewed in this series.)

Despite the fact that much of the material in the second half of the book is copied from other sources, Shi has managed to put it all together in a beneficial way. A great number of Taiji books discuss push hands and even strive to give instruction in it, but few books are entirely devoted to this aspect of Taiji. This one might not be a must-read, but it certainly is an ought-to-read.

Methods of Applying Taiji Boxing

By Dong Huling
(Originally published 1956. *Brennan Translations*, 2017, 76 pages)

Dong Huling's *Methods of Applying Taiji Boxing* is an interesting take on an Taiji applications manual. Apparently, Dong learned Taiji from his father, Dong Yingjie, and his brother, Dong Junling, acts as the attacker in the photos. (Dong Yingjie's own book, *Taiji Boxing Explained*, is reviewed in Volume VI of this series.)

The reason this manual is interesting is that it takes a Taiji form from beginning to end, with each movement depicted against an attacker. Of course, this method can only demonstrate a single application for each posture and must, therefore, leave out other possibilities—of which there are many. The form they follow is not named but appears to be Wu Family Style.

As with many Chinese martial arts manuals, this one is replete with prefaces and introductions—six including one by the author. All are similar to any other preface in any other Chinese martial arts manual, though each does deliver tidbits of information, perhaps on the art of Taiji, perhaps on push hands, or perhaps on the author's background and skill.

The main text begins with general comments on Taiji and the book that follows and includes some ancillary instructions for pushing hands.

The first text of note is copied from the author's father's book, *Taiji Boxing Explained*. It consist of commentaries on the Taiji Clas-

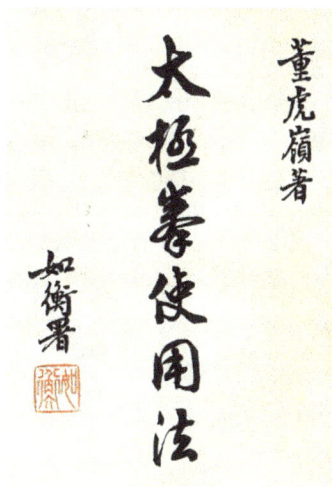

sic, *The Song of Playing Hands*. The Taiji Classics are de rigueur reading for Taijiquanists, and expert commentaries on them also are important reading. In this case, the commentaries do not stint, carrying as much weight as the Classic itself.

Next, the author dives into the instruction section for the thirty-seven-posture form. As noted before, this is a cooperative set with one person playing the attacker and the other the defender. The textual instructions are good, and the photos, while a little bland, are completely adequate. I think that this is the only Taiji manual I've seen to treat form practice in this cooperative manner.

Following the form instruction is a section depicting more applications, though this is based not on the postures of the form but on the Eight Gates: Wardoff, Rollback, Press, Push, Elbow Stroke, Shoulder Stroke, Pull/Pluck, and Split, which the author calls "Rending.". The author and his crash-test dummy go through each of them, demonstrating two additional ways to apply each of the movements.

Reading instructions and looking at photos like these might not actually teach you how to perform applications. That takes hands-on experience. But they can give you clues about how Taiji functions and about what you might want to test out on your training partner next time you meet.

PART VI

Wudang Weapons

Illustrations of Thirteen Tai-Chi Sword

by Li Zhen
(Wan Li Book Co., Ltd., 1981, 92 pages)

If you have to learn a Taiji sword form from a book, this slender volume might do the trick. I managed to learn a saber form from similar book issued by the same publisher. (See the review of *Tai Chi Tao*, by Cai Long, below.) Oddly both books have photos of the same man—Sin Man Ho—demonstrating the movements, though the names of the books' authors are different.

The text is in English and Chinese, and the expository material is limited, which probably is not a bad thing considering the awkwardness of the English translation. For example:

> The sequence requires an even and proper co-ordination in the postures and movements of the sword-fingers and the sword, so that the development from one posture into another is clearly visible, and there are no such shortcomings as paying attention to the sword-fingers but losing sight of the sword or to the upper section at the expense of the lower, and vice versa.

Comprehensible, but, whew!

Really, though, mediocre translation isn't much of an issue if you can get something from a book, and as I said, you probably

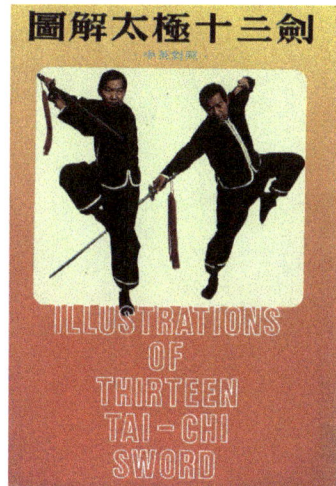

could learn a straight sword form here if you don't have access to someone to teach you.

Taiji Sword

By Wu Tunan
(Originally published by The Commercial Press, LTD, 1936. *Brennan Translations*, November 2015. 147 pages.)

I'm afraid this review is going to be very short. That isn't because I don't think this book lacks value. It certainly has value to Wu Taiji stylists who practice straight sword. And Wu Tunan was a venerable Wu sword stylist whose advice should carry weight. He was a student of Wu Chienchuan and produced a number of disciples of his own. Most of us who are familiar with him know him from photos taken when he was much older: slender as a reed, bespectacled, and white-haired with a long, flowing white beard. That is not the Wu Tunan pictured in this book. This one is a young man, whose portrait at the beginning shows a friendly and knowing smile.

The problem with this book for the average reader of martial arts literature is that the background and principles of Taiji in general and Taiji sword in particular are exceedingly brief. Perhaps the author assumed that anyone who came to this book already would be versed in Taiji history and principles. But he does give an interesting if sketchy take on the development of the straight sword and the art of wielding it, though there is a definite irony to his conclusion that students should learn a sword form—most preferably a Taiji sword form—to elevate their ability to defend their country. It

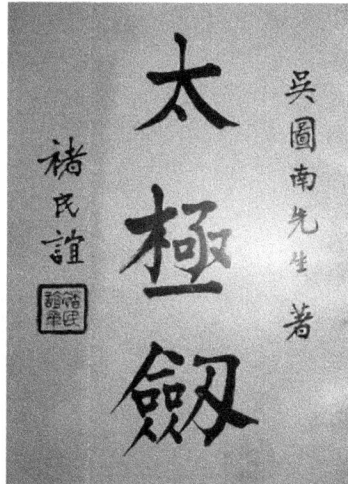

would seem that martial artists of his generation were somewhat stuck in a shadowland between a past, where the martial might of individuals might actually contribute to victory, and the future, where high-powered weapons of war virtually supplanted the edged weapons of old.

Nonetheless, its is good to have a document on Wu's sword form, for which he was apparently famous—and for which he devised the names. Except for the three pages of introductory material and a concluding chapter of just two pages that describes the general functioning of the sword movements, the entirety of the book is form instruction. Anyone who has read many of my reviews knows that I believe that such documents are virtually valueless except to practitioners of the same or similar styles or to those who desire a completist understanding of the use of any particular style or weapon. So I will recommend this book only to individuals with those proclivities. For others, there just isn't much here to grab hold of.

Taiji Sword

By Yin Qianhe
(Originally published by Pole Star Press, 1958. *Brennan Translations*,
    December 2015. 66 pages.)

Here I go again, reviewing a book on Taiji sword when I do not know much about Taiji sword, though I practiced a saber set for a brief time. But while I can't say much about the sword form depicted, I can make observations about the prefatory material. I also can say that Yin Qianhe was a notable martial artist and author of several martial arts books, some of which are reviewed in this series.

Taiji Sword is prefaced by Shen Honglie, who is described thus by the author in his own preface:

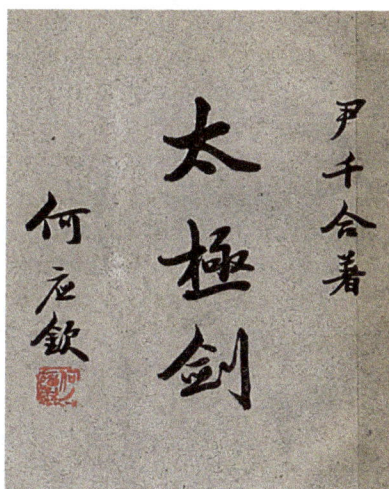

When armies were raised in resistance against Japan [during the Second Sino-Japanese War, July 7, 1937, to September 2, 1945], I followed Shen Honglie, chairman of my home province of Shandong, by serving in the army. Shen was a long-standing advocate for martial arts, so he made martial arts the major training regimen for the military, and since it is my hobby, I pursued this with extra sincerity. For fighting the enemy and smiting the invaders, it proved to be very helpful.

From this statement, we can gather that Yin's swordplay is not only sincere but actually was utilized in battle, making it deadly serious.

The second preface is by Chen Family Taiji stylist Chen Panling, who served as president of Henan Province Martial Arts Academy. Yin describes Chen by saying he received "frequent guidance from my martial arts superior, Chen Panling," among others.

To his credit, Yin provides more prefatory material for this book than Wu Tunan did for his book on Taiji sword (review immediately above). The author gives a succinct background on the development of the sword, coming to the conclusion, as have many other martial arts historians, that the background of specific martial arts—not to mention martial arts as a whole—are too hazy and steeped in myth and legend to ascertain any sort of accurate historical picture of their development.

Next is a basic introduction to Taiji sword. This includes differentiating the methodology of Taiji sword from the sword arts of external styles, distinguishing movement and stillness, coordinating the upper and lower parts of the body, and encouraging continuity of movement. This latter also takes into account the principles of sticking, connecting, adhering, and following.

The sixteen sword techniques of Yin's sword form are the subject of the next, very short chapter. They are presented as a list, each technique accompanied by a brief description of the action of the sword.

The next chapter delineates eight moral attitudes to adhere to in martial arts training. These, the author says, apply to open-hand as well as to weapons forms. As should be obvious, all are in accord with general moral principles by which most of us wish the rest of us would abide. I'll give you only the topics, though Yin provides a sentence or two of explanation:

1) Maintain seriousness.
2) Look upon others with respect.
3) Receive others harmoniously.
4) Maintain a sense of justice.
5) Practice with diligence.
6) Conduct yourself with honor.
7) Cherish compassion.
8) Give yourself with loyalty.

The final chapter before the form instruction section lays out four pointers for practicing Taiji sword. The first is perhaps the most important:

> If you wish to practice Taiji Sword, the best thing to do is start practicing Taiji Boxing.

After that, the form instruction section takes up the remainder of the book. As noted above, I'm not qualified to critique sword forms, but I will remind the reader that Yin apparently actually used a sword in combat, so that should lend some weight to the form depicted. As a final note, the sword Yin wields in the photos is quite long—much larger in relation to his body than is usually seen.

A Taiji Sword Handbook

By Shi Diaomei
(Originally published by the Huanxin Publishing Company of Taiwan, 1959. *Brennan Translations*, 2020, 64 pages)

The briefest of introductions prefaces Shi Diaomei's *A Taiji Sword Handbook*, and the entire remainder of the book consists of the form instruction section. The sixty-posture form is explicated in barely adequate text and very grainy, contrasty photos that don't always reveal the basic outlines of the movements. For straight sword exponents only.

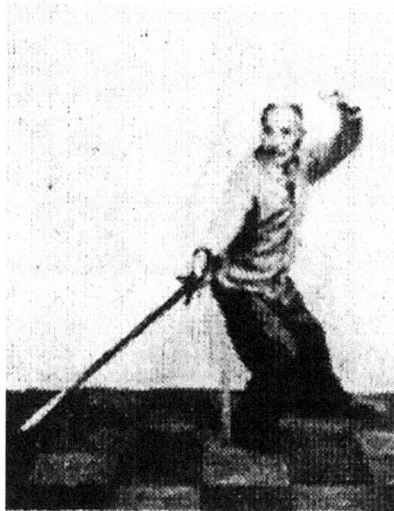

Taiji Sword
Including Taiji Long Boxing

By Chen Weiming
(Originally published 1928. *Brennan Translations*, 2012, 92 pages)

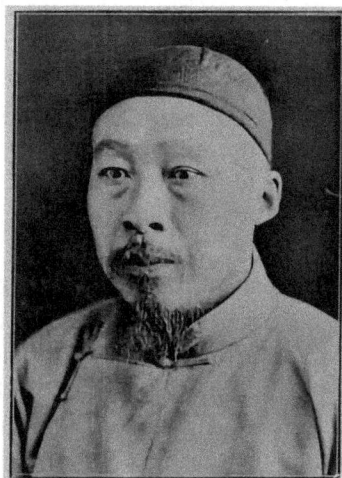

By now, readers of this series are probably familiar with the works of Chen Weiming, reputed to be one of Yang Chengfu's premier students, since I've reviewed several of his books and he also is mentioned as the author of numerous prefaces for the books of other authors. While this book by Chen contains an open-hand form instruction section, it is primarily a manual on Taiji sword, and the boxing material is secondary.

The book opens with four prefaces, the last by the author. The first one, by Qian Chongwei, relates how Qian came to study with Chen, and he also divulges a bit of Chen's background. The second preface, by Hu Puan, speaks of the sword art and its basic parameters and includes an anecdote about a bout between two swordsmen. The third preface, by Huang Taixuan, relates a bit of Taiji history linked to Taiji's philosophical concepts. Chen's own preface addresses his time with Yang Chengfu, and he also talks about some of the other masters he learned from, including Sun Lutang.

From here, the book moves straight into the instruction section, which covers a fifty-three-posture straight sword form. The textual instructions are at least adequate for this sort of material, and the photos are above average, both in size and clarity.

The next chapter contains information on the 108-posture long form as performed by Yang Chengfu. I'm not calling this a form instruction section because, although it does have textual instructions for the movements, there are neither photos nor drawing to help graphically illustrate the movements. Hence, this section should be take as simply historical material.

After that, Chen treats us to mini bios of several famous Taiji boxers, most from the Yang family, but there are a couple who aren't. These bios discuss each man's background, skill, methodology, and other aspects, including anecdotes regarding some of their martial encounters. The chapter ends with a section comprising advice on Taiji from Yang Chengfu—generally principles and precepts.

Chen Zhijin takes up the pen here for two chapters, the first on Taiji compared to other forms of exercise. These other forms are Shuaijiao, Baduanjin, Tantui, calisthenics, track and field, soccer, Western boxing, Jujitsu, and other Chinese boxing arts. Even though this material is barely more than cursory, it also is valuable and interesting for those who want to expand their comparative understanding of other martial arts.

Chen Zhijin's second chapter is on Taiji's moral qualities and functions. This text essentially states that Taiji practice imbues the practitioner with spirit and understanding, leading to virtuous, ethical conduct—not a bad place to end a Taiji book.

This manual isn't for the general reader, but is geared for those interested in expanding their knowledge of Taiji sword. However, Taiji historians could profitably peruse the list of Yang Chengfu's postures, and Yang stylists will be informed and entertained by the bios of the several Yang masters. The comparisons of Taiji with other exercise forms also might resonate with some readers.

Essentials of the Wudang Sword Art

By Huang Yuanxiu
(Originally published by The Commercial Press, Ltd, 1931. *Brennan Translations*, 2014, 78 pages)

The meat of a great number of Chinese Republican Era martial arts manuals is limited to form instruction, and that is doubly true of manuals on weapons forms. *Essentials of the Wudang Sword Art* goes beyond that limited parameter.

The book opens with a page of calligraphy that, translated, reads:

> The key in sword practice is that your body moves like a swimming dragon, never coming to a halt. After practicing over a long period, your body will united with your sword, then your sword will merge with your spirit. There will be no sword anywhere, and everywhere will be a sword. When you understand this principle, you are almost there.

Several more pages of calligraphic comments follow, leading to a mention of Li Fangchen's (Jinglin) "Magic Swords," which were twin blades carried in a single scabbard. After a portrait of the author and the man who posed with him for the form instruction photos, Huang delivers his preface. It contains a bit of his personal history, a complaint that the Japanese stole the martial arts from

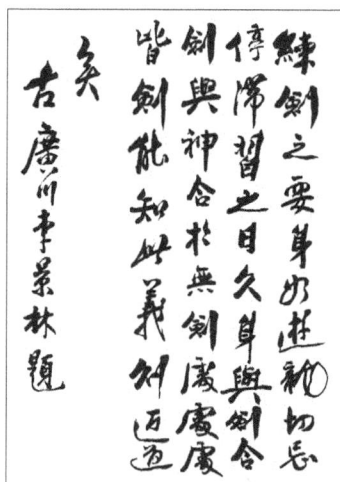

China then claimed to have invented them, and a further complaint that his own countrymen have forsaken the martial arts.

After that, Huang states the essentials of the sword art, speaking only briefly of methodology and tactics. More detail is contained in the next section, "Five Things to Avoid when Training in the Sword Art." These prohibitions—or some very like them—are stated in a great number of martial arts manuals for open-hand systems as well as weapons. The prohibitions are:

1) Lust and avarice.
2) Brutishness
3) Impatience
4) Excessiveness
5) Inconstancy

The reasons these are considered prohibitions should be obvious, even to those who don't feel prohibited at all, but the author treats each to a short paragraph of explanation.

Then he lists the thirteen techniques of the Wudang Sword art, and these, of course, are not Taiji's Thirteen Postures. They are:

1) Drawing
2) Dragging
3) Lifting
4) Blocking
5) Striking
6) Stabbing
7) Tapping
8) Flicking
9) Stirring
10) Pressing
11) Chopping
12) Checking
13) Clearing

Each of these is then explained in words and photos of the author and his practice partner squaring off with swords. As far as instructional material like this goes, this is much better than the average, really giving a sense of each movement, its dynamics, and its purpose.

Following this, which serves as the manual's technique instruction section, the author discusses Wudang Sword's hand positions modeled on the taijitu (the two-fish tai chi symbol). Translator Paul Brennan notes that these charts aren't particularly helpful, and I tend to agree.

A few words on the stages of training, from solo practice, through sparring sets, to free sparring against other sorts of weapons is next, then the author dips into two training sets: Two-Person Sword Triangles, and Passive and Active Sword Circles. After that come instructions for the Wudang Sword Sparring Set, but unfortunately, it is not accompanied by dedicated photos. Instead, the reader has to refer back to the techniques instruction section—and not in order. For example, the first movement of the two-person set requires the reader to find photos 28 and 31, movement two references photo 29, and so on, making it a confusing chore to flip back and forth and back and forth, trying to find the correct photos. And this sparring set isn't short or simple, containing five sections totaling 102 movements.

I wish you good luck in learning this set from this manual; however, the set is described more fully in *Notes on the Wudang Sword Art*, by Yi Fanzhai, reviewed next.

The next sparring set—the Lively Stepping Sparring Set—is much simpler, being only twenty-one postures long, but it is completely devoid of references to the techniques photos, assuming, I suppose, that the reader already knows what it means for "A to strike around B's wrist, then to his ear" or to perform "sweeping the hall."

The next chapter covers free sparring methods, which basically encourages the two participants to go at it as best they can, all while the sword "moves like lightning," and the body "moves like a dragon."

A couple of songs follow, one about emptiness, one about practice. After them is a short chapter on the spirit of sword practice, which takes courage, inner power, decisiveness, and an imperturbable calm. An equally short chapter on secrets of using the sword is next, and it basically encourages awareness, coordinated movement, courage, and composure.

A chapter on customized swords follows, and it discusses wooden as well as metal swords, and after that is "How to Practice the Eye Movements, Body Standards, Hand Techniques, and Footwork," which easily contains the real substance of this book aside from the techniques instruction section. Hand/eye coordination, strength, and spirit all come into play, as does practical advice on using the sword.

> The hand techniques have to do with the movement of the entire arm. Your shoulders should release downward, your elbows should adjust quickly, and your wrist should be loose but strong.

Or:

> Most will grasp the sword too tightly, a "lifeless grip." What is good about it is that you will not easily lose your sword, but it has the drawback of making you unable to wield your sword in a lively way.

In speaking of a "lively grip," the author writes:

> This grip uses the thumb, middle, and ring fingers, while the forefinger and little finger remain looser, as though the palm can hold yet a little more.

There is much more here of importance to swordplay in general, and it all would be valuable to those who undertake sword practice.

This is the end of the main text, though several appendices follow. The first is a bio of Li Jinglin, the master whose forms this book discusses. Then comes a recent lineage chart of the Wudang Sword art, a short history of the sword, and an outline of the ancient standards for making swords. This includes technical terminology, materials, characteristics, and rough dimensions. After that comes a list of fifty-nine legendary and famous swords, from one made for the Yellow Emperor all the way to the present of the book. This list ends the book.

This sword manual is definitely better than average. It has both textual substance and a generally informative instructional section that clearly shows both the movement of the sword and the purposes of those movement. Recommended for swordplay enthusiasts, but others can gain valuable information from the chapters on general martial matters.

Notes on the Wudang Sword Art

By Yi Fanzhai
(Originally published 1939. *Brennan Translations*, 2018, 48 pages)

This book can be considered an important adjunct to Huang Yuanxiu's, *Essentials of the Wudang Sword Art* (reviewed just above). It better covers the Wudang Sword Sparring Set with more thorough text and photos that might not be great but that are more than adequate. As a note, the sparring set in the other book lists five sections totaling 102 movements, while the set in this one has five sections totaling 109 postures. However, this manual contains virtually no expository material. So, combine this book with the former one, and you'll have a much more complete manual on the Wudang Sword Art.

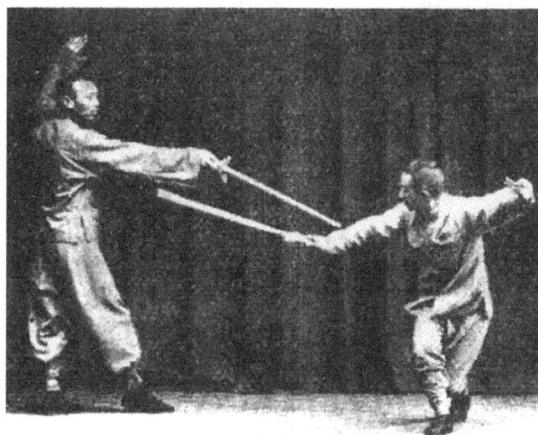

Tai Chi Tao

by Cai Long
(Wan Li Book Co., Ltd., 1980, 92 pages)

Tai Chi Tao, written in both English and Chinese, is an instruction manual on performing a Taiji saber form. It starts with a few pages that lay out basic principles, which are economically stated. Then it's on to the instructional material. The text is by Cai Long, but the photos depict Sin Man Ho.

In general, I think it's pretty hard to learn some kind of form from a book, and the instructional material in most Taiji books is somewhat weak. This book is an exception. I know that you actually could learn the saber form from it because I did. But then, I've seen a lot of saber forms—from other martial arts as well as from Taiji, so I had some sort of visual template to go by. The photos are numerous enough, and they're arranged along the tops of the pages so you get a good sense of the flow of the form. And they include plenty of arrows to indicate direction of movement.

This would be a decent choice if you want to learn Taiji saber and don't have a qualified instructor at hand. See also the review of the similar book, *Illustrations of Thirteen Tai-Chi Sword* (above), by Li Zhen but also featuring photos of Sin Man Ho. But more important, see the following review, which covers a translation of an earlier edition of the book, and the review of Tom Marks's *Tai Chi Sabre for Self-defense* in Volume II of this series.

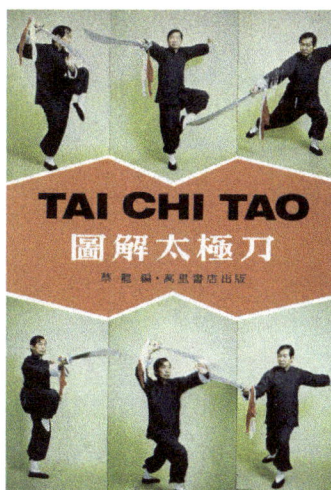

Taiji Saber

By Cai Longyun
(Originally published by The People's Physical Education Press,
    1959. *Brennan Translations*, 2014, 60 pages)

Taiji Saber by Cai Longyun is the same book just reviewed (*Tai Chi Tao* by Cai Long), in an alternate translation. The two books contain basically the same material, though there are a few differences aside from simple alterations in wording and phrasing between the two translations.

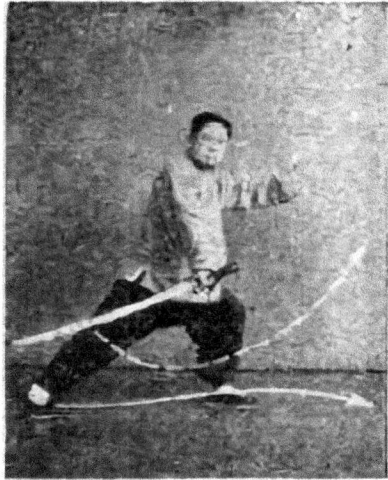

Tai Chi Tao opens with several pages of color photographs of some of the form movements, followed by ten important points and precepts to make note of, and this is followed by the form instruction section, which ends the book.

Material included in *Taiji Saber* that is not found in *Tai Chi Tao* are a short preface by Fu Zhongwen that doesn't say much, a poem on the Taiji saber, a short chapter on combat drills for two partners, and a postscript that mentions a couple of interesting points: First, the Taiji saber set illustrated in the book is only one of two the author is familiar with, the second, he believes that the Taiji Thirteen Saber set is the progenitor of the saber set detailed in this book.

And there is another, significant, difference between the two books with regard to the photos demonstrating the form. The quality of the photos in *Tai Chi Tao* are immensely superior to those in

Taiji Saber. But then, the former book was published two decades after the the first edition, and printing technology had evolved to a better state. But that isn't to say that the photos are better. The ones in *Taiji Saber* might be grainy and too heavy on the contrast, but the man demonstrating is Fu Zhongwen, the real expert here. He's the one who taught Cai and was the genesis of the book:

> Fu Zhongwen asked me three months ago to write this book for him.... At last it is finished, and I am sorry you could not be reading it sooner.

No apologies necessary, Mr. Cai. True Taiji literature is timeless.

There being little practical difference between the texts of the two editions, it's a tossup which one to peruse. I'd recommend the one from *Brennan Translations* for three reasons: 1) It has photos of the real master, even if they aren't as clear as one might like, 2) It has the added chapter on applications, and 3) It is free and readily available.

The Taiji Unfathomable Saber of the Internal School

By Wu Tunan
(Originally published by the Commercial Press, LTD., 1934. *Brennan Translations*, 2014, 98 pages)

To be clear, Wu Tunan was not a member of the Wu family that developed Wu Family Style Taiji, though he learned from the same sources as Wu Style founder, Wu Quanyu, and basically practiced Wu Style forms.

To be more specific, Wu Quanyu and Wu Tunan both learned from Yang Shaohou, who had continued to develop the small-frame Yang Style form taught to him by his uncle, Yang Banhou. This juncture between Yang Shouhou and Wu Quanyu is the seminal moment of the creation of Wu Style, and Wu Tunan was right in the midst of it, emerging as a master in his own right.

To be even more specific, here is a brief bio of Wu Tunan from the *Wikipedia* page on Yang Shouhou:

> Wu Tunan was Yang Shouhou's last living direct disciple. Born into a prominent Mongolian warrior clan in Beijing and originally named Ulabu (Wu La Bu), he was not strong as a child and so his father had him trained in martial arts. Beginning at age nine he studied the Wu style under Wu Jianquan [son of Wu Quanyu and codifier of Wu Family

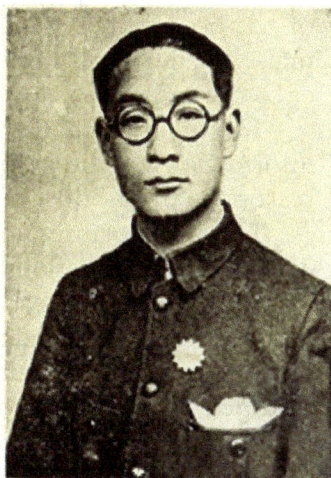

Style] for eight years, then Yang style under Yang Shouhou for four years.... Those four years were equivalent to advanced graduate training offered only to those who already had mastered the Yang large frame or the Wu style. An educator and scholar, Wu wrote extensively on t'ai chi, founded the lineage described above, and at age 100 was still performing his small frame form for the public. In the 1980s he received awards recognizing his lifelong accomplishments, and he died in 1989 at age 105.[1]

The Taiji Unfathomable Saber of the Internal School is just one of Wu's books reviewed in this series. It opens with photos of the author, prolific martial arts author Chu Minyi, and Wu Chienchuan. After that are five pages of calligraphy, some of which are examples of the book's title by the author, praise for the author by others, or praise for the martial arts. Then comes a preface by Chu and another by the author.

The first two chapters—"Generalities" and "Specifics"—include information on the author's motivations for writing the book and reasons to practice the martial arts, but little else.

The 101-posture saber form instruction section comes next. The textual instructions are okay, but the photos are pretty bad, though at least you can discern the basic postures. A concluding chapter touches on strategy and tactics, and that ends the manual.

This is simply a basic instruction manual, so readers looking for historical context, methodology, or even applications will be disappointed. But if you're into Taiji saber, you might want to take a look.

Notes

1 "Yang Shou Hou." *Wikipedia*, https://en.wikipedia.org/wiki/ Yang_Shao-hou

Tai Chi Bang
Eight-Immortal Flute

by Jesse Tsao, with Bill Coffey
(BN Publishing, 2012, 134 pages)

I can't say that I really know much about the Taiji bang, or as it's also called, the Taiji stick or Taiji ruler. At its basic, the bang is a wooden dowel, about a foot long, with rounded ends that can pivot smoothly in the palms. Author Jesse Tsao uses a length of bamboo, but attractively lathed versions can be purchased commercially. I'm a cheapskate, so I just used a rolling pin I bought at a dollar store.

I've heard the ruler disparaged as a non-classical weapon or training device, to which I say: So what? Cave men might say the same of a straight sword. If practicing with an aid, whether the stick is long or short or is wood or sharpened steel, helps you move farther along your path, go for it. I'm a non-traditionalist.

I played with the bang form Tsao presents in this book for a short while, but I dropped it fairly quickly for a couple of reasons. One was time. I already practice Taiji and chi kung, and those take enough time as it is. Lack of time, not to mention age and lack of interest, is one reason I no longer do a lot of things These might not be issues, however, for folks who are younger or more dedicated that I am. The second reason is that, after playing with Tsao's form,

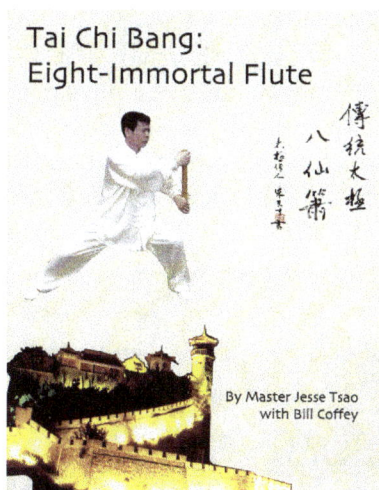

I grabbed my stick and did my own Northern Wu Style form with it, modifying the form slightly to accommodate holding the stick. So, basically, except for some of the more complex wrist twisting movements, you can create a ruler form out of your own already familiar Taiji form.

This isn't to say that Tsao's book has no value. Anybody who's seen Tsao's application videos on *YouTube* knows he's pretty good at Taiji. The book lays out his ruler form quite clearly, and it's easy to follow. Another nice point is its reference to the Eight Immortals. A lot of us have noticed images of these mythic Chinese figures here and there, but Tsao presents five pages containing mini-biographies of them. Nice.

And to go back to the criticism that the short stick isn't a classical weapon—well, maybe not. But that doesn't mean that it can't be used effectively. There's a nifty martial arts scene in the otherwise lackluster movie titled *The Island* (1980) in which a karateka armed only with a belaying pin, which is about the same size and configuration as a bang, defends himself against a sword-wielding modern-day pirate. The pirate eventually wins (by cheating, of course), but the episode shows how effective a bang can be, even against a sword.

Chinese Wand Exercises

by Bruce L. Johnson
(William Morrow & Co., Inc., 1977, 220 pages)

Sometimes, the story behind a book is as interesting as the book itself, and in the case of Bruce L. Johnson's *Chinese Wand Exercises*, both hold considerable interest. I'm going to treat the book first, leaving the back story for last.

Chinese Wand Exercises discusses the background, philosophy, principles, and methodology of a series of bending and twisting exercises performed with a bamboo stick—or, wand—that is about four feet long. At present, at least in English, there are only two books on these exercises: the one under consideration and a more recent volume by a British Taiji teacher named Michael Davies. I haven't yet seen Davies' book, but in on-line material, he states that he learned the exercises from Johnson's book. Davies is now one of the premier disseminators of these exercises, which are sometimes call by other names, such as Taiji wand or stick exercises.

I can see how Davies could learn wand work from Johnson's book. The text and graphics for the instructional section are clear and well-defined, and the exercises themselves are relatively simple and straightforward. In his introduction, Johnson lays out the basics:

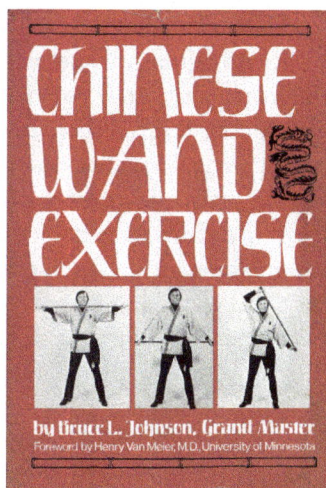

With this Wand one goes through a series of movements specially designed to get the blood circulating and recirculating more efficiently throughout the body.

The purpose of using a wand, he says:

[is that] it is your tangible and your security, giving you just the right amount of resistance needed to complete the movements. The Wand maintains your balance and provides you with perfect form and posture.

Wand exercises, Johnson informs us, go back thousands of years. Originally, they were developed as an exercise routine for Chinese royalty, and the methodology was, for centuries, a carefully guarded secret. From his brief history of wand exercises, Johnson segues into a discussion contrasting internal and external exercise arts that would not be out of place in any Taiji book. In this discussion, he draws on the concepts of yin and yang and chi energy, distinguishes limitations people might have in practicing, and points out the ways that modern society sabotages health.

The first chapter relates how Johnson learned wand exercises, but I'm saving that for later. Instead, we'll move on to chapter two, which the author uses to give a short background for the wand art, focusing mostly on a sort of philosophical history that mentions Taiji and acupuncture. Chapter three, also short, goes into yin and yang theory and chi energy in succinct detail.

Chapter four describes what Johnson calls the "Element Stage System." In short, the exercises advance through a specific progression of intensity, each stage represented by one of the Five Elements of Chinese philosophy: wood, water, fire, air, and metal. The idea is somewhat complex and not fully expanded upon until a couple of chapters later.

Correct breathing is the subject of chapter five, and after a general discussion of breathing, Johnson explains the concept of deep breathing, for which he gives a specific formula for advancement. He then moves on to meditation breathing, again with a specific formula to follow. The way to breathe during the wand exercises is next, and after that, he talks about what he calls "combination breathing," which is breathing through the nose and mouth at the same time. None of this is abdominal breathing, per se, but the techniques are pretty good nonetheless.

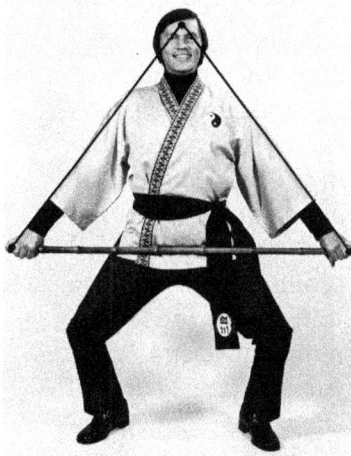

The wand itself is the subject of the next chapter, which covers the ideas behind the wand, including a sort of "triangulation effect" that the exercises promote, which causes the body, when holding the wand, to arrange itself in a three-point structure. This triangulation produces what the author refers to as "pyramid energy," and I notice that the tantien is almost always one of the points of the pyramid, and when it's not, the tantien is usually situated at the center of the pyramid's base, as in the photo above. The chapter also talks in general about the physical makeup of the wand.

Chapter seven relays information on advanced meditation techniques to assist the practitioner in working through the Element Stage System. A thirteen-page Q&A chapter comes after, and it covers just about any question you might normally ask about wand exercises, from whether it can affect weight loss to details on the techniques involved.

The next chapter contains the fundamentals of wand exercises, such as grip, positions of the wand, and stances. Until now, there have been no illustrations, but from here on, almost every aspect of what the author talks about is illustrated with large, clear photos, and some intriguing drawings.

The wand exercises themselves occupy the last two-thirds of the book. There are seventeen of them, though Johnson claimed that he knew 190 more, some that produce esoteric effects. The exercises progress from the simplest to the more difficult, but none of them are what might be termed strenuous or complex, though they might grow more intense.

Each exercise is explained in very clearly detailed text that leads off by pointing out which muscles are involved and then talks about the process of passing through each of the five elemental stages while going through the movements. And because of Johnson's five-stage system, they can be performed in a large range of intensities.

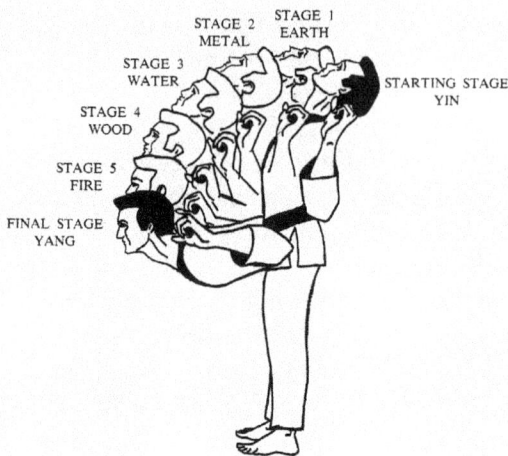

The text for each exercise is accompanied by three types of illustrations. The first are straightforward photographs showing Johnson in the beginning and end postures. The second show the same photos with straight lines drawn from point to point of the triangular structure, as in the photo on the preceding page. When the movement is more complex, additional photos, also with the triangle defined by lines, describe the basic movements between the beginning and end postures. The third type of illustration is one that, to my knowledge, is unique to this book.

These are line drawings by Joel Rogers, one of Johnson's students, that vividly portray the exercises' movements. Most of us are familiar with photos in which a moving subject is lit by a strobe light, resulting in a photo that depicts several stages of a movement within a single frame. That's what these drawing do, handily portraying the entire range of each exercise's movement clearly defined within Johnson's five-stage system. Some include overhead views in addition to a front or side view to fully expose, if necessary, the movement's dimensionality. Really, if you can't learn to do these exercises from these instructions, don't blame the book.

I've long believed that one of the great benefits of Taiji as a physical exercise lies in the way it exercises muscles by twisting and extension rather than by clenching and compression. And those are just what the wand exercises in this book do. Heck, I feel better just looking at the photos! I have to admit that I never seriously undertook these exercises, but having revisited the book, I find myself inclined to try them out again.

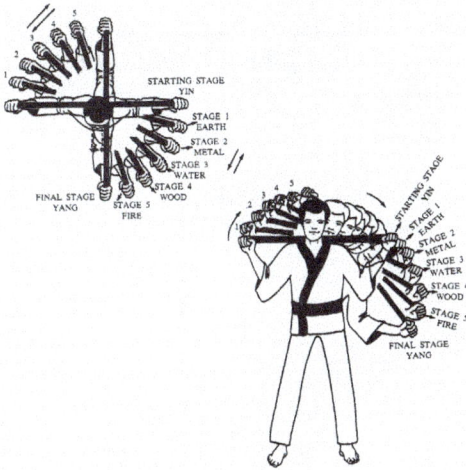

All-in-all, this is a very worthwhile book: well written, informative, and containing something useful that is well explained. But if you're interested in learning these exercises from a book, you might have to pass on this one. *Chinese Wand Exercises* only enjoyed one hardbound and one paperback edition, both published in 1977, and not only is it out of print, used copies are quite expensive. I did find one copy of the hardbound on sale for $40, but after that, the prices ranged from a low of about $150 to a high of nearly $2,500! The cheapest paperbound I saw was $50. I picked up my hardbound copy in a used bookstore in about 1980 for less than $10, and, wow, I now see that it's actually autographed by the author! Not only that, but I also have the bamboo wand that came with it. Do I hear $3,000...?

So, for those who are interested in learning these exercises, you'll probably have to go with Michael Davies' book, *Jiangan: The Chinese Health Wand*. As I said above, I haven't seen Davies' book, but my understanding from the book blurb is that it contains all seventeen of the exercises that Johnson depicted in his book.

Now, it's time to get to the interesting story behind the author and his book, though parts of it are, perhaps, suspect to one degree or another.

Bruce L. Johnson was quite a guy, though his end was less than desirable, from a kung fu standpoint. Ironically, his background, though American, could be the story of any number of kung fu greats: sickly child overcomes

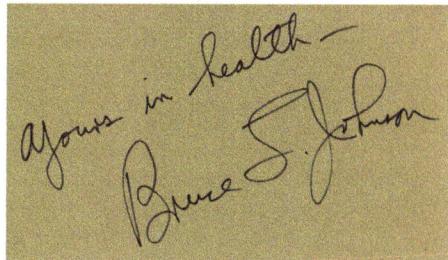

his weak beginnings through exercise and body-building to become a champion.[1] While serving during WWII, Johnson won the Navy heavyweight wrestling championship. He also was one of the first to land on Iwo Jima. After the war, he earned three black belts in Judo in Japan.

Subsequently in Shanghai, he and a couple of buddies, who also were Navy wrestlers, were being ridden around town by an eighty-year-old rickshaw driver. The Americans were amazed that the old man could easily haul their three beefy frames up and down hills with ease, and Johnson asked his secret. In response, the old rickshaw driver took him to meet a tall, slender, and regal ninety-three-year-old Chinese man referred to only as Dr. Ch'eng. Johnson says that Ch'eng looked to be about fifty. And, luckily for Johnson, he spoke perfect English.

One of the first things Johnson noticed about Ch'eng's well-furnished home was the great number of four-foot-long bamboo rods, or wands. Some were polished and carved with elaborate designs and others were embossed with metal. The wands, Ch'eng told Johnson, were used for an esoteric exercise system of which Ch'eng was the grand master. Each of the wands in his home represented one of his pupils, who possessed an identical wand.

Ch'eng looked pretty fit to Johnson, who was not then aware of the old man's true age, but the American couldn't understand how waving a stick around in the air could provide a thorough exercise. Eventually, after a number of meetings during which they discussed kung fu and Ch'eng ascertained the quality of Johnson's character, he asked Johnson "to come at him with my strength, and all that I knew." The burly American, already a third dan in Judo, was reluctant to attack the slender old man, but Ch'eng insisted, so Johnson complied.

Johnson writes of the results:

> Suddenly, before I had made contact with him, I felt something like a wind, a gentle but firm pressure on me from a "breeze"…but I was experiencing this strange sensation while seated on the floor!

Ch'eng was just standing there, smiling and looking as if he'd never moved. Ch'eng asked him to repeat the test two more times, each time with the same result. Ch'eng had, he explained to Johnson, learned the "art of spinning" from his father.

Johnson writes:

> One must, have perfect balance, agility, and coordination to turn around in a tight circle so fast that the human eyes watching do not detect any movement at all and even a trained observer sees only a blur of movement.

Johnson says that Ch'eng could spin once to repel a single attacker or several times in the case of multiple attackers. Ch'eng then taught Johnson his secrets. His own sons had been lost in the Sino-Japanese War, and he entrusted Johnson to carry the art, with integrity, into the future and into the world.

It's a very neat story. Do I believe it? Shrug. I wasn't there, so I don't really know. But Dr. Ch'eng's "spinning art" seems suspiciously like Taiji, though Johnson doesn't call it that. In addition, Chinese wand exercises often have been referred to as Taiji stick or wand exercises, so that strengthens the potential link between the two arts.

Johnson promptly tried to introduce wand exercises in the United States but failed due to the fear of anything Asian fomented by McCarthyism. Gradually, though, as that era passed, Americans became more receptive. In the mid 1960s, Johnson taught wand exercises to a number of famous people, including Mae West and Jimmy Durante, and became friends with Bruce Lee and actor James Coburn, who was pictured on the cover of *People Magazine* doing a wand exercise. Johnson said that he and Lee would give demonstrations of strength and speed, and he claimed that, aside from Dr. Ch'eng, Lee was the only person he knew who could best him.

While on a trip to the Bahamas in 1965, Johnson was at the beach when four children swimming in the water were attacked by a shark. Johnson rushed into the water, pausing only to grab the one weapon he could find, which was a large seashell. The shark killed one of the children, but Johnson fought it off while the others escaped. The shark grabbed Johnson by the leg, and he fought it off by gouging out one of its eyes with the shell before staggering back to the beach, bleeding profusely. According to the *Wikipedia* article on Johnson, there are about fifty other documented cases of Johnson risking his life to save others from dangers that included fires, mangled cars, and even abusive husbands. Heck, I'm in my seventies, and I haven't even been around that many life-and-death situations, much less been the hero of them.

Apparently, the esoteric kung fu Johnson learned from Dr Ch'eng lent Johnson a sort of mystical power.

> Students would sometimes notice supernatural transformations in his appearance [that made him appear to be an old Chinese man] as he taught the class. He was inclined to believe that Dr. Ch'eng was teaching through him. One famous psychic of his day, Peter Hurkos, upon meeting Johnson reportedly said, "Who is that beautiful Chinese man coming out of you?"[1]

By 1976, Johnson was working as a professional diver, when an accident left him with a near-fatal brain stem infarct causing stroke-like symptoms. The doctors told him he'd never walk again, but he was moving around again in a few months. The next year, he published *Chinese Wand Exercises*. To tell the truth, he looks pretty damn fit in the photos, not like a man who nearly died the year before. And he doesn't look fifty-one, either. But maybe that's because of the big smile that spreads across his face in almost every photo—a smile, by the way, that really looks like the man is happy, confident, robust, enjoying what he's doing, and relishing life.

But as I promised above, Johnson's end was not so benign. I can't pretend to understand the forces at play. Maybe the spirit of Dr. Ch'eng finally abandoned Johnson, leaving him to the wiles of a popular culture in which the born-again Christian movement was beginning to rise. Johnson found Christianity, and a Christianity of the variety that considers chi power to be the energy of Satan. He later said:

> These things are not from God, as God is not in the business of mystical energies or the occult. I no longer practice the martial arts.... As a Christian, I cannot in good conscience, teach or recommend the martial arts to others.[1]

I might argue otherwise, both about what we think we know about God and about what these energies actually are—certainly not Satanic—but Johnson will never hear me. He died in 2014, leaving his book containing seventeen wand exercises with us but perhaps taking 190 more to the grave.

> I am the last of the grand masters [of the Chinese wand]. When I go, the secret goes with me.[1]

Others, as I mentioned above, however, are resuming Johnson's work—notably Michael Davies. We don't have those missing 190 exercises—at least not in the public forum—but maybe one day they will be rediscovered. Until then, Johnson's book, being the sole definitive text on Chinese wand exercises, will have to stand as the Taiji Classic of the art. It deserves to be reprinted.

Afterword

As with a couple of other of my reviews, readers have responded with additional information. The following is edited from an an email exchange with Peter Zoll, who also teaches these wand exercises and has done some background research on Johnson.

> I managed to get Bruce Johnson's high school yearbooks and his U.S. Navy service records. He looks pretty scrawny in the former, and his enlistment documents have him as 5'10" and 142 pounds. How much time, if any, he could have spent ashore in Shanghai is hard to determine. He never mentions the names of anyone in the crew who might have been with him.
>
> Actually, I have to admit that I like some of the exercises and actually teach them. More importantly, my students like them. To be fair, they may just be enjoying me struggle with some of the behind the back sections. To Johnson's credit, some of his exercises cover muscles that the World Health Qigong Yangsheng Zhang routine does not.
>
> I paid for copies of all his service records. They are pretty sparse—there is no mention of any athletic achievements. He served on the seaplane tender *USS Norton Sound* from

January 1945 to June 1946, but we are talking seventy-five years ago, so I was not surprised that the webmaster did not think anyone was still alive from that time. As you may know, Johnson was in the Navy from June 1944 to June 1946. He did not last very long at the University of Minnesota. Here's what the official history of the ship has:

> After Pacific shakedown, the new seaplane tender stood out from San Diego 26 February 1945 and steamed for Pearl Harbor, Hawaii. She reported for training in mid-March, and she arrived Saipan 1 April 1945 to provide seaplane tending services. (Note that Ernie Pyle was killed April 18 1945 at Iejima.)[2]

> *Norton Sound* anchored 1 May 1945 at Aka Kaikyo, Kerama Retto, and by 21 June 1945 had assisted in downing three hostile air raiders. Air alerts continued until midnight, 14 August 1945. Word of the Japanese surrender arrived eight hours later, and into September the tender engaged in upkeep and air operations at Okinawa.[3]

The ship steamed for Sasebo, Japan, September 21, 1945, returning to Okinawa one week later. *Norton Sound* called at Shanghai, China 1 October 1945, and by the 23rd of that month she was at Tsingtao, where she tended seaplanes until November 7, 1945. About three weeks at Shanghai. November 8, 1945, she anchored at Shanghai, and from then until April 1946, she remained on duty with the occupation forces between China and Japan.

Could Johnson have gotten shore leave? If so, long enough to learn wand exercises? He may have had a chance to get ashore during the second "tour" when the *Norton Sound* spent more time there later. Still, the logistics of getting leave and going ashore for significant periods are daunting.

Norton Sound departed Tokyo Bay 7 April 1946 for Norfolk, Virginia. After overhaul there she joined the Atlantic Fleet. She operated off the east coast until October 1947, when she steamed for San Diego to rejoin the Pacific Fleet.

1936 to 1976 or so is a very tough period to get accurate (or sometimes any) historical documentation from China. Still, as you indicated, how hard could it be to give the master's full name and address? Johnson might have wanted to send a postcard saying he arrived back in the U.S. safely. Or to ask about a post-war visit. And if there were other bamboo wands, there must have been other students—but there are zero names of other students.

I would like to think that there are some true stories somewhere in his history, but I would be inclined to give him credit for the exercises and leave it at that.

In Chen Family Style Taiji Chuan, double batons (sometimes known as maces) is a canonical set. As far as I know, only Grandmaster Chen Zhenglei and Chen Ziqiang have recorded the set. But the batons are double and 26" long versus single and 48" for the wand.

The World Health Qigong set is somewhat similar to wand although it features movements in one set as opposed to seventeen exercises

Casting a wider net (outside the internal martial arts) there's the whip stick from Tong Bei and the Japanese jo. The sticks there are shorter and the movements make up one set.

How privy Johnson's widow was to all this is not clear. I'd be interested if anyone else has any comments. I would have thought that Johnson would have had at least one disciple in all those years who got the full system. If so, he or she has been very quiet.

Notes

1 "Chinese Wand Exercise." *Wikipedia*, http://en.wikipedia.org/wiki/Chinese_Wand_Exercise

2 https://www.history.navy.mil/research/histories/ship-histories/danfs/n/norton-sound.html

3 From https://www.history.navy.mil/research/histories/ship-histories/danfs/n/norton-sound.html

PART VII

Narratives

Secrets of the Tai Chi Circle
Journey to Enlightenment

by Luke Chan
(Benefactor Press, 1993, 134 pages)

Most people who write about Taiji and related arts do so from instructional or philosophical standpoints. They relate the history, philosophy, and principles of the art, and they demonstrate a form and perhaps a few applications. Some dedicated authors go on to discuss the dynamics of Taiji and other more complex subjects. There are few Taiji book, however, quite like Luke Chan's *Secrets of the Tai Chi Circle*.

Secrets of the Tai Chi Circle is not an instructional or expository text. It's a short novel that follows the life of a young man as he discovers and learns about Taiji in conjunction with discovering and learning about life. The setting is China—in proximity to Chen Village—but the time frame is never precisely defined, seeming to be any time prior to the 20th century. Along the way, the young protagonist finds puzzles and answers, love and sorrow, and loss and attainment.

There are no rousing fight scenes here. This is a Taiji novel in the same way that Mark Salzman's *Iron and Silk* is a kung fu novel (and, later, a movie), though Chan's book is not as directly autobiographical. But while it is short on action, it is long on philosophy and filled with vignette-style episodes that attempt to convey the meaning of Taiji in a sincere and more realistic way than does the

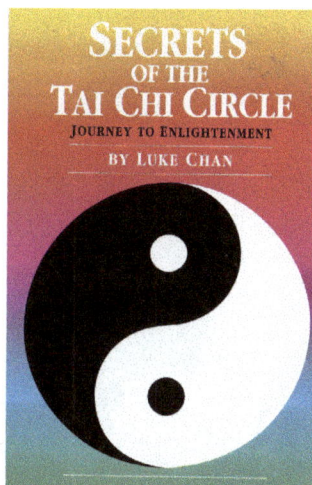

average kung fu story. After all, the lives of most of us are not informed by mystic monks and punctuated with combat but are strewn with the daily vicissitudes that give us all plenty of trials and tribulations to deal with.

I'd call this a philosophical book, and I liked it overall, though I confess that it sometimes seemed facile, maybe because some of the vignettes were familiar to me from elsewhere. It's not a book that will teach you much about doing Taiji, but it will help you learn how to apply the principles of Taiji to everyday life, and that's a pretty good endorsement. It's also a pleasant read.

Laoshi
Tai Chi, Teachers, and Pursuit of Principle

Laoshi's Legacy
Emergence from Shadow

by Jan Kauskas
(Via Media Publishing, 2014, 184 pages, 2018, 220 pages)

Most books on Taiji and other martial and movement arts are didactic in method—they are, to a greater or lesser degree, textbooks that define the parameters of the art they describe. They generally discuss the fundamentals and principles of the art in question, and many attempt to define their art in terms of history, social norms, scientific and engineering principles, or philosophy, including ethics as well as meaning and spirituality. A great number also include an instruction section that features illustrations and written descriptions of how to perform the movements of the art and how to apply the movements in combat. Sometimes these are well done, sometimes less so. I delineate martial arts books into three categories:

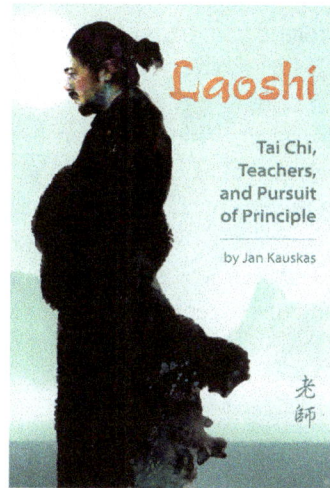

1) Those that contain basic background and philosophy, working methodology, and form instruction;
2) Those that usually eliminate form instruction in favor of greater emphasis on the more purely historical or philosophical;

3) And those that emphasize fundamentals, principles, dynamics, or specific methodology.

The first sort of book is geared to the beginner and intermediate student, while the other two types are more for the intermediate and advanced student, though beginners often can benefit from them. *Laoshi: Tai Chi, Teachers, and Pursuit of Principle* and *Laoshi's Legacy: Emergence from Shadow*, by Jan Kauskas, are examples of the third sort. The two books form a sort of yin/yang Taiji dynamic, the first book emphasizing the student/teacher relationship and the second the teacher/student relationship. In the first, the student learns Taiji from a teacher, and in the second, he learns how to be a teacher of Taiji. As becomes evident over the course of the two books, these two aspects are at the core of Taiji's continual generation and development.

The Laoshi books are not didactic exercises that discuss Taiji in terms of movement, martial applications, history, or philosophy. Instead, they employ a method not usually seen in martial arts literature, though parallels can be found in the basic question-and-answer sessions that one sometimes sees in Taiji books. One excellent example is *T'ai Chi Ch'uan Ta Wen: Questions and Answers on T'ai Chi Ch'uan*, by Chen Weiming. (See review in Volume V of this series.) In these Q&A sessions, students ask questions of the master, whose answers are sometimes straightforward, sometimes cryptic. If you haven't read such a book, you probably should, though surely you've seen many kung fu movies in which the young acolyte asks questions of his or her teacher during training, who, often as not, responds with fortune-cookie philosophy.

But the *Laoshi* books are more than a Q&A. Instead, they comprise what is essentially an extended Socratic dialog between a student and his teacher that unfolds over more than two decades and that strives to find the heart of Taiji rather than to parse its details. Such a dialog goes beyond mere Q&A, into the realm of conversation, in which instruction and talk are followed by rumination and practical examples that are followed, in turn, by more conversation and more rumination. Consequently, the books dip into a structural and stylistic territory that is fresh for Taiji books and offers an organic method of delivering in-depth information.

This is not to say that the *Laoshi* books are novelistic in approach. Although martial arts novels abound in the East, to my knowledge, there is only one Taiji novel in English: *Secrets of the Tai Chi Circle: Journey to Enlightenment*, by Luke Chan. (Reviewed above.) While that book bears some of the same hallmarks of Socratic dialog as the *Laoshi* books, it remains novelistic in that it follows a narrative to tell a story that has a plot in addition to the explicit and implicit Taiji instruction. The *Laoshi* books, though they do utilize a methodology that is more novelistic than the typical instructional Taiji text, are plotless and too picaresque to be novels in the strict sense. Kauskas simply calls them a semi-fictional memoir.

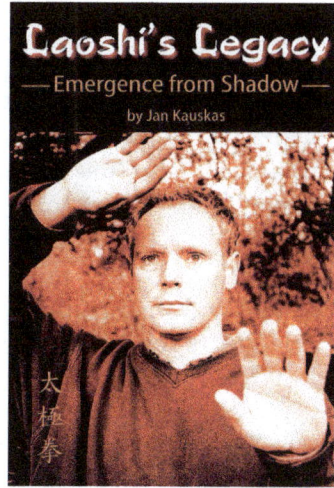

Laoshi tells the story of an unnamed Taiji player, loosely based on Kauskas himself, who I'll call Student because, after all, he's not actually Kauskas. After studying several martial arts other than Taiji with various teachers and masters, he becomes a student of Laoshi. The name Laoshi has often been attributed to Cheng Man-ching, but the character of Laoshi is not a real person or based on one. Instead, he is an amalgamation of various teachers and masters Kauskas studied under. The word means "teacher" in Mandarin, and as Kauskas puts it:

> "[Laoshi represents] the best aspects of the many martial artists, whose skills dedication, and wisdom inspired me in my attempts to match their example.

And often, other teachers Kauskas mentions also are amalgams, perhaps including the character of one of Laoshi's instructors: Wang Lang. Wang's genesis in these books is unclear to me, but if he is fictional, he is appropriately named since there actually was a Wang Lang who lived during the Northern Song Dynasty (969–1126). This historical Wang is considered to be one of the most important martial arts masters of antiquity for his creation of Praying

Mantis kung fu. Some teachers named in the *Laoshi* books, however, are—or were—real people, notably Billy Coyle, an Aikido expert who pioneered that art in his home country of Scotland and who died in 2011, and the aforementioned Cheng Man-ching (Zheng Manqing), who was one of Laoshi's principal teachers and whose Taiji style and philosophy permeate the book.

The first book opens with Student just beginning his study under Laoshi, who he calls "the real deal, or at least as real as it gets these days." (An ironic statement since Laoshi is a fictional character!) The first paragraph begins:

> I'm not sure I like Laoshi, my teacher. I'm not sure he likes me. I'm not even sure you are supposed to like your teacher.

Like each other or not, these two form a long-lasting and ever-deepening student/teacher bond whose history progresses through the course of the two books. Along the way, Student's learning experiences, whether gained in a martial arts studio or on the streets of daily life, lead him to ponder the nature of the martial arts, Taiji, life, and the nature of reality and to pose questions on those and other subjects to his teacher. Laoshi almost always answers—usually warmly—in the arcane manner of every archetypal martial arts master you've probably seen in hundreds of martial arts films.

Relentlessly wise and experienced, Laoshi is the teacher we all wish we'd had. Although some of his answers are as boilerplate as those of kung fu film masters, that isn't necessarily a detraction. Any practitioner of the martial arts or reader of martial arts literature is going to be familiar with most of the principles, fundamentals, and philosophy contained in these books because they are built into this arena of human endeavor. It is the personal nature of the narrative that makes those principles, fundamentals, and philosophy live, breathe, and speak deeply to us.

But most of Laoshi's responses to Student's questions are too acute and involved to serve as chopsocky metaphors, and in the end, their occasional familiarity doesn't detract from their basic profundity, which often is enhanced here by specific dilemmas or circumstances surrounding a given question posed by Student. A diamond, in other words, can look no better than cut glass unless it's surrounded by a setting that helps focus attention on refractions of the gem's heart.

Another minor detraction is that the Socratic dialog occasionally seems forced. For example, well into Student's apprenticeship—and after he's taken over Laoshi's teaching duties—he has an exchange with Laoshi during which Laoshi explains the paradoxes of the maxims from the Taiji Classics: "My opponent moves, but I move first," and "Attack and defense are simultaneous." I don't quibble with Student's finally "getting" these paradoxes internally. That's what this book is about: discovering something, parsing it, and finally internalizing it. But until he finally starts wondering about these specific matters, he seems to have been completely ignorant of them, which is inconceivable in any advanced practitioner. These are among the basic self-defense concepts of Taiji and are spoken of frequently in the literature. Did Student never read the Taiji Classics?

But such is the nature of the Socratic dialog, in which students ask questions of the master that range from the profound to the profoundly obvious and dumb. The point is not literary realism but to relay knowledge and understanding. Still, Student's ignorance in this area at such a late date in his training should have required a set-up that doesn't exist in the exchange. But perhaps I quibble, and to be fair, the discussion of the topic proceeds to unfold over the course of many pages into a flower of significant depth and breadth, finally revealing the essence at its core.

Unlike most Taiji literature, the *Laoshi* books do not deal with Taiji dynamics, per se, or even form. The two principal Taiji-specific topics the author explores are push hands and swordplay, and the books would be especially valuable to readers with those same interests—and to students of Cheng Man-ching's Taiji, for there are many references to Cheng and his main students. But for Taiji players of other styles, there is plenty of practical information, ranging from discussions of the angle of the torso to thoughtful words on the potential legal complications that can arise from using martial arts in a real-life situation. And Student's quest to become more learned as well as more expert in Taiji opens up meanings that apply beyond both dynamics and form and extend to life itself.

The narrative, such as it is, is not a straightforward rendition of Laoshi's teachings and Student's progress. It follows the general progression of Student's apprenticeship, but throughout are asides, flashbacks, and reminisces in which both Laoshi and Student relate martial arts experiences—some gained from the time before their teacher/student relationship, some gained together. For Student, this brings in Billy Coyle, and for Laoshi, Cheng Man-ching and Wang Lang, among many others. Late in *Laoshi's Legacy*, Laoshi tells Student:

> If a successful taijiquan teacher is one with many students, then that success is not built on skill or teaching ability alone. It often comes down to who can tell the best stories.

This might be so. Instruction can elucidate principles, but stories bring principles to life. Instruction is the form, describing and delineating, while stories are push hands, illuminating the interplay of life's shifting energies. In fact, the pages of both books are replete with concepts, stories, and quotations that the canny Taiji instructor might profitably borrow to more greatly inform his or her own students' practice.

So there are lots of asides, segues, and anecdotes to keep the texts of the two books moving in a literary rather than a didactic fashion. This is important to the books' success, both in delivering information about Taiji and in developing an approach to the art that helps further one's practice on multiple levels—not just the physical, but the intellectual, emotional, and spiritual. In other words, these books are not just a dry reads—which isn't necessarily bad—but are immersive and refreshing swims in the great Taiji river.

In the final analysis, Jan Kauskas has produced a pair of very fine books on Taiji that remind us that learning and teaching Taiji are not just about taking in or imparting the movements of a form, experiencing the interplay of push hands, or dealing with the mechanics of weapon play. It is as much about our connections to life and to the Tao. More than anything, the *Laoshi* books reveal both the ever-evolving nature of the art of Taiji and the evolution of the martial artist.

The Wandering Taoist

By Deng Ming-Dao
(Harper & Row, 1983, 240 pages)

It's reasonable to assume that most readers of this book will have a basic knowledge of the teacher/pupil relationship within the martial arts and of the young martial artist's journey from a state of powerless ignorance to one of greater skills and understanding. This motif—defined by mythologist Joseph Campbell as the "Hero's Journey"—features in literally countless martial arts films, sparked by Chinese Wuxia (martial heroes) novels bearing similar tales of personal development. In drama, often the motivation is revenge, but in Deng Ming-Dao's *The Wandering Taoist*, the motivation is a combination of cultural continuity and personal development for the purpose of spiritual advancement and elevation.

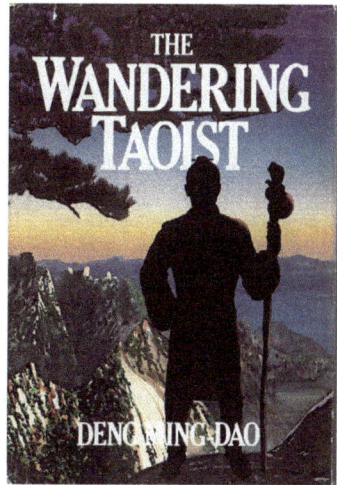

Deng Ming-Dao is a Chinese American author, artist, philosopher, teacher, and martial artist specializing in the internal martial arts and chi kung. He is the author of several other books and is a fine artist and graphic designer whose work is in several collections, including the Brooklyn Museum. From a young age, he studied martial arts and chi kung under a couple of masters before studying with the subject of this book, Taoist master Kwan Saihung, for thirteen years.[1]

The Wandering Taoist is a biography of Kwan, from his birth into a family of nobility, through his years of rigorous education and training as a Taoist acolyte, to his enlightenment and reentry into the world as a wandering Taoist unconnected to a temple, although he remains a member of Taoism's Zheng Yi sect.

Kwan—whose family name was originally Guan—was born in 1920. The large household was overseen by his grandfather—a strict but also kind man also expert in several martial arts, which he taught to the young Kwan, who was an unruly and headstrong child. Eventually Kwan was sent off to a Taoist monastery to complete his formal education in the Five Excellences: Traditional Chinese Medicine, calligraphy, painting, poetry, and the martial arts.

The expectation of his family was that, once he reached a certain level, Saihung would return to the fold to contribute to the family welfare and continuity, but as willful as ever, Saihung decided to continue pursuing Taosim by formally becoming a monk. For this act, his grandfather ostracized him and told him never to return. Saihung had little choice but to remain at the temple and resume his studies and esoteric practices.

Saihung tells many stories, but one that sticks in my mind concerns Yang Chengfu. In Saihung's account, he and his mentor met with Yang on a street, and just moments later, Yang was attacked by three men intent on doing him harm. According to Saihung, Yang killed all three in short order while he and his mentor watched.

Saihung's training proceeded for a few years until the outbreak of the Second Sino-Japanese War, upon which Saihung, consumed with nationalistic fervor, left the monastery along with a couple of other acolytes to join the army in its attempt to repel the invaders. For this, the monastery's Grand Master ostracized him and told him never to return.

Saihung fought in battles for several years, but finally, exhausted, he left the front and returned to the temple, where he discovered that the Grand Master had forgiven him. Not only that, he told Saihung that it was time to complete his studies by undergoing the ordeal of remaining sealed for months in a maze of caves. Inside this warren, Saihung is confronted by several demons who attempt to lure him from the Taoist path. The book ends with Saihung's epiphany and the Grand Master leading him from the darkness.

This summary merely skims the surface of the story, which is purported to be a straightforward biography. It was well written and interesting to read, though is sometimes seemed like a massive cliché of the hero motif, complete with monsters and demons, though the battles with them do not involve weapons other than the spirit, will, and mind.

While this is supposed to be an accurate account, there are a few jarring instances that seem to be awkward at the least, and illogical at worst. One occurs close to the end of the book, when Saihung is in his mid to late twenties. Until this point, he has had an excellent education in the Chinese Classics through his grandfather and his years of study at the Taoist monastery. He has read the Classics and memorized a number of them. Yet after all of that, right before Saihung is shut up in the cave, the author states that the Grand Master introduced him to the *I Ching* and taught him about the hexigrams. Really? I'm not even Chinese, and I first heard of the *I Ching* when I was about twenty-two. I find it inconceivable that Saihung had to be "introduced" to it and have it explicated for him this late in his life. The book is a Chinese cultural icon, and surely he would have known of it much sooner—perhaps since childhood.

This may be a quibble, but less so is the fact that Saihung came from a family that could afford every opportunity for leisure and learning the martial arts. They had servants to take care of their needs. He was, in short, a rich kid who had all the advantages in life and who eventually excelled. I'm much more impressed by the disadvantaged kid who makes good despite the tremendous obstacles in the way of advancement.

Despite this, the book was a pleasant read, and even the more fantastic elements, such as the demons and some of the martial actions, are in keeping with a journey toward enlightenment. I can't say I learned much, but I did find some validation.

Notes
1. "Deng Ming-Dao." *Wikipedia*, https://en.wikipedia.org/wiki/Deng_Ming-Dao.

Encounters with Qi
Exploring Chinese Medicine

By David Eisenberg, M.D.
With Thomas Lee Wright
(W.W. Norton & Co., 1985, 254 pages)

In 1971, an article by columnist James Reston appeared in the *New York Times* relating his experience when he accompanied Richard Nixon's entourage to Beijing. While there, he was stricken with acute appendicitis. Apparently, he underwent the surgery to remove the appendix without chemical anesthetics, the only palliative being "acupuncture anesthesia."

Prompted by this astounding reporting, Dr. David Eisenberg made several trips to China, from 1977 through 1985, to study acupuncture and the energy of the human body known as "qi," "chi," "ki," "prana," and numerous other names. Indeed, he was the first Western physician to visit China in an attempt to study this energy in concert with physicians of Chinese Traditional Medicine (TCM) of various sorts, chi kung experts, and even Chinese doctors trained in Western medicine.

Perhaps "study" is too strong a word. What Eisenberg is doing is taking a low-altitude survey of the qi landscape to get the lay of the land and to verify that, at least, there are headwaters and reservoirs of chi. So this isn't a book about research, but rather about Eisenberg's encounters with many people who can alter chi flow

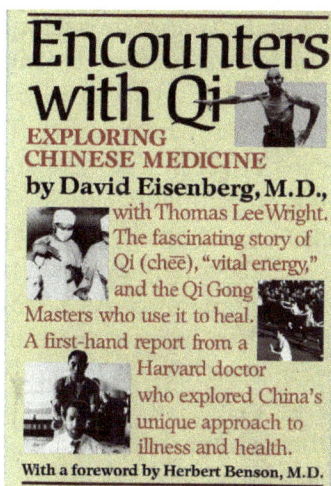

(physicians) or generate it (chi kung masters and several others with innate abilities).

During his time in China, Eisenberg didn't just observe. He obtained training in various TCM techniques, and as the first Western doctor to do so, he was introduced to a number of qi experts—both medical and others—and shown a number of demonstrations of the power of qi, including the moving of inanimate objects, the lighting of florescent light tubes through touch alone among others. The collection of individuals he met was diverse, but the real shame is that among them there were no high-level Taiji masters who also could externally express internal energy—this despite the fact that Eisenberg says he practiced Taiji during much of his stay in China.

Eisenberg begins with a chapter recounting his early months in China and how he acclimated—and how his Chinese neighbors and colleagues reacted to him. For most, he was the first Westerner they'd met. He also introduces Dr. Fang, who began teaching him Chinese medical theory. There are many details in this chapter that I can't cover in a review, so suffice it to say that Fang's discussions of the components of TCM are interesting and germane to the practice of, especially, the internal martial arts.

Particularly eyeopening for Eisenberg was Fang's discussion of human anatomy. As a Western-trained physician, Eisenberg was well versed in human anatomy—or thought he was until he was faced with the Chinese version of anatomy which is more akin to an energy matrix of esoteric "channels" that carry the "vital fluid" of qi throughout the body. So, first, Fang had to teach him what "qi" is—at least in general terms since nobody seems to truly know what it actually "is."

The discussion of chi and its generation naturally leads to a section on qi gong masters, which also entails a definition of qi gong. Eisenberg describes several types of qi gong and masters who could perform seemingly amazing feats. Part and parcel of all this is the background of Chinese culture and governmental rule, the latter which in the form of the Cultural Revolution, oppressed practitioners of qi gong and Chinese martial arts, driving them underground. Fortunately for Eisenberg, by the time he arrived in China, the sway of the Gang of Four had dissipated, and the government was once again fostering the qi arts, though in a tightly controlled manner.

The next chapter goes into some of the nuts-'n-bolts of Eisenberg's training. First, he had to learn to diagnose the patient from careful observation of the tongue. While Western physicians tend to downplay the relationship of the tongue to various physiological states, TCM utilizes tongue diagnosis as its first-line tool. As Eisenberg puts it:

> There are thousands of permutations and diagnostic combinations. A comprehensive medical education includes the study of hundreds of tongues....Patients suffering from serious illnesses had tongues deviating from the normal color, texture, shape, and coating. Expert doctors of traditional medicine were able to predict the form of the tongue, without even seeing it.

Diagnosis from the pulse is covered next. This isn't the single pulse that Western medical practitioners feel, but rather six in each wrist, three of them somewhat deep. Eisenberg writes:

> Doctors study pulses for frequency, rhythm, strength, volume, and other characteristics. They use terms like *floating*, *slippery*, *bolstering-like*, *feeble*, *thready*, and *quick* to describe clinically the nature of the pulse. An abnormal pulse corresponds to a specific bodily imbalance.

And, in keeping with the practice of physicians everywhere, there is the patient interview, and it is here that the cultural differences between the East and West become very apparent. While Western doctors ask open-ended questions in an attempt to draw out the patient and get them talking about their problems, TCM physicians ask direct questions. And these questions can be very different from those asked by a Western doctor. From this, Eisenberg segues into a long section on the methodology of medical diagnoses, comparing and contrasting Western medical practices with TCM.

Acupuncture is the subject of the next chapter, and the author goes into some detail on the historical background of acupuncture, his training in it, and some of the positive effects that he saw acupuncture produce. After a month of theoretical training, he went on to work in a clinic under the supervision of a master acupuncturist. The training included, of course, understanding of the meridian system and the many acupuncture points along its channels. It all begins with Eisenberg receiving a needling from his instructor so that he knows how it feels to have the needle inserted, but more importantly, to feel the sensation of "obtaining qi." This is the sensation of qi build-up at the insertions point.

There is a great deal of controversy surrounding acupuncture, but Eisenberg discusses many obvious—if still-mysterious—effects of acupuncture, beginning with acupuncture analgesia. This is the very topic that prompted him to study TCM, and he discusses a number of specific case—among many—in which sometimes serious operations were successfully carried out using only acupuncture as a painkiller. He goes into some of the reasons that acupuncture might have this pain-killing effect but also says that much more serious research needs to be carried out to understand the underlying mechanism.

Then he moves on to what I might call the "gee-whiz" chapters, beginning with his meeting the Wang sisters who could accurately identify to contents of a box merely by touching it. He was lucky to have had the opportunity to meet them because, as he puts it, these sorts of innate abilities are considered Chinese state secrets. Despite Eisenberg's initial skepticism, the sisters accurately described whatever he or the colleagues who'd come with him put inside the box.

This experience led Eisenberg to seek to study a high-level qi gong master, but that had to wait as he continued his acupuncture training and took up therapeutic massage. He recounts the conditions of several patients with different maladies, some of whom were helped and some of whom weren't. Notably, one or two weren't helped because they weren't really sick. Call them hypochondriacs.

Eisenberg's training in herbal medicines comes next. Do these herbal concoctions actually work? Sometimes maybe not, but Eisenberg relates the story of a young man who, on the outside was a beefy weight-lifter, but who was suffering from ulcerative colitis and experiencing intense intestinal cramping and pain. After the usual tongue and pulse examinations, the doctor wrote out a prescription of nine herbs with which to make a daily tea. Eisenberg writes:

> In a Western medical facility, the evaluation and management of this patient would have been entirely different. He would have had blood tests and an extensive physical examination....

He probably would have been hospitalized immediately and treated with antibiotics and other medications. His doctors would also have considered surgery, particularly since ulcerative-colitis patient who do *not* have their colons removed face a significant risk of developing colon cancer.

But the doctor who wrote the prescription told the patient:

> Your condition has been studied for hundreds of generations. The prescription I have written for you was recommended by the famous Dr. Li Shi-jen in the year 1578 and is still the most effective.

Was it effective in this case? Apparently. When the man returned a week later for a follow-up, he proclaimed that the cramping, pain, and bloody diarrhea had subsided within three days of taking the herbal concoction. By the end of the week, all the symptoms had vanished.

The next chapter relays Eisenberg's encounters with masters of qi gong. He writes:

> Qi Gong masters were considered state secrets in 1979. In that year Beijing's "democracy wall" was dismantled and numerous Chinese were imprisoned for sharing "state secrets" with foreigners. Some of my colleagues were eager to satisfy my curiosity about Qi Gong masters, and I feared that this might cause them political trouble.

Nevertheless, Eisenberg did meet with several chi gong masters who performed a variety of feats for him, including breaking rocks with bare hands and moving inanimate objects apparently with qi alone. He also met with researchers who were studying chi gong masters and their abilities. You'll have to read the book, however, to get the gist of what the researchers had learned.

A lengthy discussion of the various types of doctors practicing TCM in China follows. Eisenberg writes:

The role of the classical Chinese physician, unlike that of most Western M.D.'s, was to teach patients to maximize health by living correctly.

Eisenberg not only discusses the parameters of being a doctor of TCM, he brings in the words of several TCM physicians to elucidate not only their roles within Chinese society but their training, as well. This training was not consistent over the course of the 20th century, and the author describes the training TCM doctors received at various times, both with explanatory text and with the actual words of doctors trained at these different time. The picture has not always been pretty, and even now the Chinese people are suffering due to poor management of the healthcare system.

Those who suffer most, perhaps, are those with mental illnesses, as detailed in the chapter that follows. According to Eisenberg, at the time of the writing of this book, mental illness was largely ignored as a mental condition or imbalance. Instead, TCM—and Chinese culture as a whole—tend to consider mental illness to be an imbalance of bodily functions—in short, an imbalance of qi. Well, this might be so, and it might not be so. Only further development of the medical and psychological sciences will determine that. But in the interim, the Chinese people are left with a society that tries to downplay the role of mental illness and subsume it within the same category of illnesses as ulcerative colitis. The chapter details a number of encounters Eisenberg had with patients exhibiting neurotic to semi-psychotic behaviors for which the TCM doctors prescribed acupuncture and herbal treatments. As Eisenberg states, many of these patients return week after week with the same complaints, yet they and their doctors seem blind to the fact that their conditions remain statically bad.

The next chapter concerns both demonstrations of qi and scientific research into this elusive energy. Some of the research Eisenberg mentions has produced positive results for the medical community. Acupuncture, for example, has been established as an effective anesthesia, at least for some surgeries. It and qi gong also have a meliorative effect on a number of other human ailments, such as high blood pressure. But he doesn't excuse the sometimes slipshod research techniques of the Chinese researchers at the time.

More carefully designed experiments need to be performed to accurately suss out the truth behind qi.

The chapter continues with qi gong as practiced by masters in public classes. This entails a lengthy discussion on qi gong in its various types, but it is in no way an instructional text, merely descriptive. The final chapter, "The Marriage of Chinese and Western Medicine," bemoans the fact that the two systems of healthcare management seem so diametrically opposed. But his belief is that each of them has something to offer the other, and that a blend of the two traditions would create a stronger gestalt.

Encounters with Qi is an interesting read, and not only for its information on qi and the state of research into the phenomenon in China. It also provides a glimpse into Chinese culture and also the machinations of an authoritarian state determined to control an energy not ameliable to external control. The only real drawback is that the information is now nearly forty years out of date, and undoubtedly much more careful research into qi has been done in the interim.

Tai Chi
The True History & Principles

Lars Bo Christensen
(Lars Bo Christensen, 2016, 152 pages)

This book isn't really a narrative, but the other books in this series were completed before I ran across this volume, and this was the only place left to put it. But in a sense, it is a narrative of Taiji history, so I'll have to be content with that.

Taiji was almost completely unknown outside of China even in the year of my birth, which was 1950. Now, slightly more than seventy years later, it, along with other Asian martial arts, has exploded within the world consciousness. Can anyone not almost totally isolated, either geographically or culturally, not have heard of Taiji? It's that slow-motion martial art and exercise....

Following not long after the explosion of Western awareness of Taiji came questions about it that went beyond how the form flows and functions and the role of internal energy in the equation. These were questions about Taiji's historical foundations. Surely such an excellent physical and kinetic art cannot simply have appeared as if divinely inspired—though truthfully, most of the streams of the several internal martial arts have headwaters in the Wudang Mountains, among divinely inspired Taoist anchorites. Surely Taiji has an actual history of progressive development from rudimentary forms of martial arts.

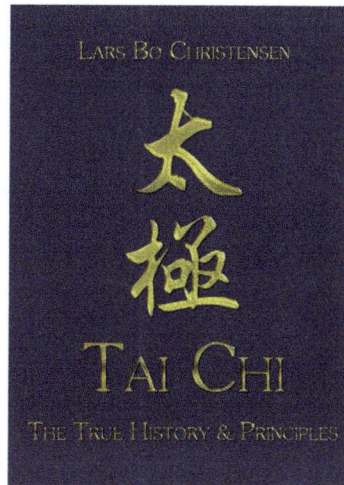

For decades, the only story regarding the genesis of Taiji told in the West was the tale of the Taoist monk Chang Sanfeng. Already trained in Shaolin-style martial arts, Chang was in a position to benefit from witnessing a confrontation between a crane and a snake. Despite repeated efforts by the crane to jab or grab the snake with its beak, the snake's sinuous coiling evaded the blows and, in the same moment created opportunities for the snake to counterstrike. This demonstrated that flexible, coiling movements were superior to sharp, linear movements in defeating an enemy. That night, an ancient versed in martial arts appeared to Chang in a dream and taught him the rudiments of Taiji spear.

After awakening in the morning, Chang began to develop systematic internal style movements, creating a rudimentary Taiji form that he then passed on to others. During the several centuries that followed, subsequent students of Chang's soft style of boxing further developed the physical techniques and chi kung aspect, and the art eventually met up with a principal exponent, Wang Tsung-yueh. Wang was reputedly an itinerant martial artist who made his living teaching in some town or other them moving on to the next. He also supposedly wrote some of the earliest works on Taiji, and his writings rank highly among the Taiji Classics. One of Wang's students was Chiang Fa, and according to the standardized history, either Wang or Chiang taught Taiji, then simply called the Thirteen Postures (Dynamics, etc.) or Long Boxing for the length of its practice set, to Chen Wangting in the middle of the 17th century.

The Chen family disputes this, claiming that Chen Wangting created Taiji on his own, basing it on external martial arts he already was familiar with. The problem with this is there is no real precedent for Chen to have suddenly discovered Taiji on his own. In fact, circumstantial evidence for his having learned from either Wang or Chiang includes the Taiji practiced at Zhaobao Village, which has its own and very old version of Taiji. Zhaobao Taiji is very similar to, but not exactly like, Chen Taiji, and Zhaobao tradition has it that they learned it from Wang at about the same time that Wang taught it to the Chens.

From the Chen clan onward, Taiji history is relatively clear and straightforward and not often disputed. What is disputed is Taiji's murky past prior to its advent in Chen Village, and historians have found more than the single and admittedly flimsy strand of transmission represented by the Chang Sanfeng story. In fact, a great number of Taiji manual from the Chinese Republican Period—1912 to roughly the end of World War II—cite five or six stories regarding the inception, development, and transmission of Taiji-like internal martial arts. These several strands, they say, culminated in the cluster of arts we know as Taiji and several additional internal arts with Taiji-like principles, such as Liuhebafa (Water Boxing). Even some modern authors ascribe to the "various strands" theory. (See the Appendix at the end f this volume for a list of books and manuals reviewed in this series that contain versions of the "several-strand" theory or even alternate Taiji histories.

With *Tai Chi: The True History & Principles*, Lars Bo Christensen enters into this arena with a sound take on Taiji history based on a relatively recently discovered group of texts that have proved to be some of the oldest extant Taiji writings. These were found in the *Li Family Martial Arts Manual*, and they were written by members of the Li family of Tang Village in Henan Province., who learned the art in the Thousand Year Monastery, located in their village. Christensen writes:

> This art may of course have been inspired from an even older tradition, but the texts of the *Li Family Manual* prove with great certainty that Taiji as we know it was transmitted from the Thousand Year Temple in Henan Province…. The Li family texts provide us with the oldest known principles of Taiji, and they are an invaluable source to determine how the art was originally practiced.

Christensen's aim with this book is to translate the new material from the *Li Family Manual* and use it and other sources to suss out the development of Taiji in those early years—and, in the course of things, he strives to pinpoint Chen Wangting's introduction to the art that was soon to define his entire clan.

Christensen opens with a chapter discussing Taiji literature, from the oldest known—the Taiji Classics—to more modern books on the art. Involved in this is the notion of the development and refinement of Taiji literature over time, particularly of books and manuals written in China during the Republican Era. This material is sketchy but germane, and a few tidbits of Taiji lore are strewn among the sentences.

A history of Taiji comes next, and this is where Christensen comes into his own with a discussion of the discovery of the *Li Family Martial Arts Manual*, which was hidden in the home of a member of a branch of the Li family that no longer practiced Taiji. The possessor was initially very reluctant to show the document to others, but after he was convinced to do so, their importance and value became clear. The manual was hidden along with a number of other old family documents, including deeds and a family genealogy written in 1716 but going back to 1590. The martial arts manual contained material dated between 1590 and 1787. The first texts that relates to. Taiji were written more than 400 years ago by Li Chunmao.

It might seem that the martial arts manual texts are the most significant part of this cache, at least in terms of history. One of them, titled, "Treatise of the Health Preserving Boxing System of the Endless Void," describes the boxing system developed by Li Daozi, abbot of the Thousand Year Temple. Two others are titled, "Poem on the Practice of the Thirteen Movements," and "Treatise of the Thirteen Movements." But as important as the Taiji texts are, the Li family genealogy is perhaps more important because it lays out a direct transmission of Taiji during an enormous blank period in Taiji history.

The genealogy makes clear that Li Chunmao learned this early Taiji system at the temple under the Li Daozi, who also was known as Monk Ten Powers. Chunmao's two sons also studied the art at the temple, and alongside them was their cousin, Chen Wangting. Yes, *that* Chen Wangting. The chapter continues with brief bios of subsequent Li family Taiji experts, but perhaps the most significant aspect is the assertion that the Li family documents prove that Chen Wanting did not invent Taiji, as the Chen family claims, but that he simply learned it along with others at the Thousand Year Temple. Notably, Taiji's reputed founder, Chang Sanfeng, is absent from the Li accounts of Taiji's transmission. But if the Li family records are accurate, then Li Daozi is the first person historically known to have practiced Taiji and passed on the art in a traceable path of transmission to the Chen family.

Unfortunately for us, no one in the Li family still practices Taiji, so we can't see what it was that Li Chunmao and his immediate successors practiced. But undoubtedly, it was very similar to early Chen Style since both sprang from the same root. Indeed, in this account,

Wang Tsung-yueh was not a major link in the Taiji chain descending from Chang Sanfeng to the Chen family, but was a student of Li Chunmao's grandson, Li Helin. Furthermore, the Li's hometown of Tang Village and the Thousand Year Temple were only twenty miles from Chen Village, also putting both in geographic proximity to Zhaobao Village.

The brief snipped of text that follows these revelations concerns the name of the art of Taiji. Originally called the Thirteen Movements (Postures, Dynamics) or Long Boxing, it is specifically named "Taiji" in a text written by Li Helin, dated 1787. Christensen acknowledges, however, that the term might have been in use in the temple before its public revelation. In fact, one of the buildings at the temple is called the Taiji Temple.

Next comes a chapter on the writings of Chang Naizhou (1736-1795), who also lived near Chen Village. Chang left a body of texts about his internal boxing system, the principles of which are clearly similar to Taiji. Christensen writes:

> Chang Nassau's writings contribute to confirm that there was a broader culture of internal martial arts in this area of China.... However, because we now have the Li Family genealogy and martial arts manual, we know that the main reason for the similarities is simply that Chang Naizhou was also studying martial arts with Li Helin.

Christensen continues with short takes on Chen Style, Yang Style, Wu/Hao Style, and Zhaobao Style—other styles, such as Wu Family, Sun, Song, and so forth, are not covered in this book. Each of these first four offshoots is linked as branches to the main trunk of the Taiji tree. For those who are curious, Chiang Fa makes an appearance as a student of the Li lineage and later was probably the progenitor of Zhaobao Taiji.

Christensen's main task is to translate the *Li Family Martial Arts Manual*, but before that, he translates a stele written by Pu Guan in 1716. This text speaks of the life of Li Daozi and makes the claim that he "was the original founder of the superior system of the Health Preserving Boxing System of the Endless Void."

Following this, Christensen presents a new Taiji family tree, with Li Daozi at the top, followed by Li Chunmao and, subsequently, his sons, Chen Wangting, Li Helin, and Wang Tsung-yueh. The family tree then descends into the familiar territory of the Chen, Yang, Wu, and other Taiji styles developed and refined over a period of several centuries until modern times.

A sketchy but useful timeline of Taiji history comes next, beginning in 67 C.E. with the founding of the Thousand Year Temple in and moving on to Li Daozi's creation of the earliest form of Taiji in about 650. The history then takes a radical jump to 1716 and the writing of the stele, and on through the subsequent development of Taiji up until 1933, when Chen Xin wrote the first book on Chen Style.

Then it's on to the main feature: Christensen's translations of the Taiji Classics of the *Li Family Martial Arts Manual*. He begins with an essay on the parameters of the Classics and, after comparing the Li family's versions with others already in the public sphere, concludes that the Li family texts are older. Part of his analysis is textual, in which he sees in all the later versions alterations in the core language that don't exist in the Li family manual, leading him to conclude that all the later versions were copies in which the copiers made errors in their transcriptions or introduced errors in meaning. All of these *Li Manual* Classics were written by members of the Li family, principally Li Chunmao and Li Helin, but a couple of them, in slightly altered versions, have heretofore been attributed to Wang Tsung-yueh. If Christensen is accurate, then Wang should be considered a talented student of Taiji who helped further the art, not as the author of any of the Taiji Classics.

The Li Family Manual texts, as are all of the Classics, whoever wrote them, are relatively short pieces filled with pithy statements on Taiji's theory, principles, actions, and dynamics. There are fifteen Classics, including those usually attributed to Wang Tsung-yueh, three of which concern weapons (saber, lance, broadsword). Much of the material in these Classics will be familiar to readers, other aspects less so, but in either case, Christensen's translations are excellent, and the texts are worthwhile reading for any Taiji exponent.

After presenting these newly found Classics, the author pens a chapter on the philosophy of Taiji. This begins with an examination of the taijitu as an enduring philosophical metaphor for the nature of forces at play in the universe. Some of his discussion is historical, some philosophical, some practical, and he brings in quotes from notable Taiji exponents and other sources from the past, such as Yang Chengfu and the *I Ching*, to bolster his argument.

The discussion continues by examining the influence on the taijitu and Taiji from Neo-Confucianism, and later Chinese philosophical writers, and it eventually touches on the yin/yang dichotomy and, briefly, the Five Phases, which Christensen says is a more appropriate translation for the Five Elements.

The author's look at Taoist influence on Taiji begins with definitions of qi (chi), jing (internally stored energy), and shen (spirit), but the discussion is brief though cogent.

Traditional methods of training Taiji is the subject of the next chapter. He starts by contrasting Taiji training from training in qi gong and hard-style fighting systems. The notions here aren't new or especially revelatory, but it's always beneficial to review Taiji's principles and methodologies.

A section on the Thirteen Movements (Postures, Dynamics, etc.) follows, and Christensen points out that they aren't really postures but are dynamic movements. In this section, Christensen has a different take on several of the Thirteen Movements than are usually elucidated, and his somewhat detailed dissection of the movements help to prove his points. The use of the voice—an aspect of Taiji that I've almost never seen discussed in books or manuals—finds expansion here beyond the simple "Heng, Ha" vocalizations used in some Taiji ancillary exercises.

Push hands is covered only briefly, but the discussion does include a translation of a text by Yang Banhou that talks about push hands. This text seems rather mild considering Banhou's reputation for harshly treating his students. After this, Christensen presents lists of the names of the movements of Taiji sword, Li Family Style, Chen Style, Yang Family Style, and Wu Yuxiang Style.

All of the above material fills the first half of the book, but the latter half of the book is almost empty of text, being occupied, first, by photo reproductions of the *Li Family Genealogy* and the *Li Family Martial Arts Manual*. There are captions to explain what you're looking at, but all the writing is in Chinese, so unless you can read that, you'll find nothing more to peruse for the next eight pages. But of course, you've already read the translations. After that, Christensen fills the remainder of the book with illustrations and photos. One of the illustrations is a 19th-century map of Yongnian, the village where Yang Luchan lived in proximity to the Wu family. A few pages containing photos of more Chinese text lead to sixteen pages of portrait photos of significant Taiji luminaries and a handful of other shots. The luminaries are featured in high-quality full-page photos that really do justice to their countenances in a way that other Taiji books have not generally managed to replicate. Of similarly high resolution are a couple of pages of Yang Chengfu in the the Taiji postures Beating Tiger and Brush Knee Twist Step.

A couple of additional pages of photos of Chinese book covers and pages finish the illustrations and photos section and lead to what Christensen titles, "Overview of Old Tai Chi Texts." This is a ten-page chart with five columns. The first column gives the Chinese title to the text, the second quotes the first line of the text, the third the author, the fourth the versions that have appeared in early Chinese-language texts and books, and the fifth names English translations that exist, if any. This chart might be useful if you wish to personally translate and compare your translations with others, or if you simply wish to compare and contrast the differing versions, particularly with regard to the Li family texts, which Christensen considers to be the originals. Otherwise, this chart will not divulge any additional information to the casual reader.

Taiji: The True History & Principles is a worthwhile addition to Taiji literature in English and goes some way in clarifying Taiji's transmission, though it really doesn't clear up all the murk surrounding Taiji's early development. Christensen seems convinced that Li Daozi created Taiji, but he largely relies on the writing of a man who lived more than a thousand years after Li died. Did Li truly create Taiji, or did he simply pass on what he'd learned from someone else? Or was he merely one among many who were creating internal martial arts that led to Taiji? After all, there are numerous other strands of Taiji history that, while not negating Christensen's take, provide alternate avenues of transmission of internal styles.

While I enjoyed taking in Christensen's history—and learned a lot in the process—I have to say that this book is a bit disjointed. Each chapter is a narrative, but the book as a whole seems choppy in construction, and I sometimes wished that Christensen had done another edit or two for style, syntax, and structure. But these are minor points for those seeking information, which Christensen clearly delivers. Recommended.

Appendix

Histories of the Genesis and Development of Taijiquan

Histories of Taijiquan that go beyond the Chang Sanfeng narrative can be found in these books, all of which have been reviewed in this series. However, in the reviews, I have generally made no attempt to parse or even discuss these histories beyond mentioning them. For a closer examination of these histories, the reader should consult the actual works, listed below in alphabetical order by author's family name. The volume in which each book is reviewed is shown in parentheses.

Chen Weiming—*The Art of Taiji Boxing* (Volume VI)

Chen Zhenmin & Ma Yueliang—*Wu Jianquan Style Taiji Boxing* (Volume VI)

Chen Ziming—*The Inherited Chen Family Taiji Boxing Art* (Volume VI)

Christensen, Lars Bo—*Tai Chi: The True History & Principles* (Volume IV)

DeMarco, Michael—*Chen Tai Chi* (Volume II)

Docherty, Dan—*Tai Chi Chuan: Decoding the Classics* (Volume V)

Dong Yingjie—*Taiji Boxing Explained* (Volume VI)

Gu Ruzhang—*Taiji Boxing* (Volume VI)

Huang, Wen-shan—*Fundamentals of Tai Chi Chuan* (Volume V)

Huang Wenshu—*The Skills and Essentials of Yang Style Taiji Boxing* (Volume VI)

Jou Tsung Hwa—*The Tao of Tai Chi Chuan* (Volume V)

Li Shoujian—*Descended from Wudang: The Taiji Boxing Art* (Volume VI)

Long Zixiang—*A Study of Taiji Boxing* (Volume V)

Lu Shengli—*Combat Techniques of Taiji, Xingyi, and Bagua* (Volume IV)

Smith, Robert W.—*Chinese Boxing: Masters and Methods* (Volume III)

Song Shuming—*The Taiji Art* (Volume VI)

Tian Zhenfeng—*Taiji Boxing Explained* (Volume VI)

Tseng Ju-pai—*Primordial Pugilism* (Volume VI)

Wan Laisheng—*Original Postures of Taiji Boxing Explained* (Volume VI)

Waysun Liao—*Tai Chi Classics* (Volume V)

Wong, Doc Fai & Jane Hallander—*Tai Chi Chuan's Internal Secrets* (Volume V)

Wong Kiew Kit—*The Complete Book of Tai Chi Chuan* (Volume V)

Wu Tunan—*A More Scientific Martial Art: Taiji Boxing* (Volume VI)

Xiang Kairan—*My Experience of Taiji Boxing* (Volume V)

Xu Yusheng—*Taiji Boxing Postures Explained* (Volume VI)

Xu Zhiyi—*Simple Introduction to Taiji Boxing* (Volume V)

Yao Fuchun & Jiang Rongqiao—*Taiji Boxing Explained* (Volume V)

YMCA Taiji Boxing Club's Anniversary Book (Volume V)

Phosphene Publishing Company
publishes books and DVDs relating to literature,
history, the paranormal, film, spirituality, and the
martial arts.

For other great titles, visit
phosphenepublishing.com

www.ingramcontent.com/pod-product-compliance
Lightning Source LLC
Chambersburg PA
CBHW060049100426
42742CB00014B/2755